Chair Yoga

Accessible Sequences to Build Strength Flexibility

(Challenge to Lose Belly Fat Sitting Down with Low-impact Exercises in a Day)

Marshall Taylor

I0089822

Published By **Darby Connor**

Marshall Taylor

Chair Yoga: Accessible Sequences to Build Strength Flexibility (Challenge to Lose Belly Fat Sitting Down with Low-impact Exercises in a Day)

ISBN 978-1-7751012-1-5

Legal & Disclaimer

The information contained in this book is not designed to replace or take the place of any form of medicine or professional medical advice. The information in this book has been provided for educational & entertainment purposes only.

The information contained in this book has been compiled from sources deemed reliable, and it is accurate to the best of the Author's knowledge; however, the Author cannot guarantee its accuracy and validity and cannot be held liable for any errors or omissions. Changes are periodically made to this book. You must consult your doctor or get professional medical advice before using any of the suggested remedies, techniques, or information in this book.

Table Of Contents

Table Of Contents

Chapter 1: Chair Yoga

Chair yoga is a derivation of the traditional yoga exercise that includes poses that pass decrease returned over 5000 years in the beyond. Most —if now not all— of the poses found in traditional yoga poses are replicable for chair yoga.

The chair yoga concept changed into coined due to the fact we spend masses of time sitting at our desks or touring from one area to three one of a kind, so why now not maximize the enjoy thru assignment a motion which can help boom flow into an exercise in our each day normal.

The identical manner the body moves thru the float of movement and will increase flexibility whilst carrying out traditional yoga, chair yoga additionally lets in actualize this. In addition to improving your variety of motion, the huge workout known as pranayama (additionally referred to as respiratory techniques) within chair yoga allows create spatial attention. It furthermore lets in you exercise meditation and reduces tension.

As the call shows, you perform chair yoga from a sited, snug characteristic. That is why the exercising is right for the disabled or the aged who are too antique to get up or exercising without hurting themselves. It is likewise first rate if you are affected by conditions like osteoporosis, continual ache, and more than one sclerosis.

The essence of the chair is to make sure you stay robust and don't stress your middle as an awful lot on the equal time as doing the sports. Therefore, if you discover the traditional yoga exercise too traumatic or tedious, you have to attempt chair yoga that will help you acquire all of the blessings of the exercise.

But in advance than we're able to start looking at the severa chair yoga practices to be had as a manner to attempt, permit's first test the severa benefits of chair yoga.

The Benefits Of Chair Yoga For Seniors

Traditional yoga poses have tested powerful at coping with numerous highbrow and bodily issues. Since chair yoga is a model of the standard yoga exercise, the blessings are more likely the identical, if no longer higher, particularly if you're a senior who can do nearly all the poses from the consolation in their seat.

Some of the outstanding advantages you stand to gain from chair yoga encompass:

Helps in building power

Any hobby that includes using your muscle mass allows make more potent them as well. Therefore, each time you have interaction in yoga poses on the consolation of your seat, numerous muscle groups carry out the interest, which allows assemble power. Therefore, this means that the extra you have interplay in a single-of-a-kind yoga practices, the greater muscle strength you assemble.

When you bring together your electricity, you furthermore may improve your balance which can be very vital in stopping falls. Additionally, the more muscle tissues you construct, the greater energy you burn and the more bone density you benefit, making every day sports lots much less complex.

Helps in ache manipulate

Most of the ache we experience, particularly as seniors whilst doing numerous sports activities, consequences from the muscle tissue not being strong or bendy sufficient to cope with the pressure. Since those yoga practices assist beautify the power and electricity of your muscle companies, you'll maximum likely no longer experience any pain at the same time as doing the sports.

This practice is also important for people affected by ache-associated situations like arthritis. It gives you severa techniques collectively with deep breathing, mild movement, and controlled visualization that help you deal with the pain and pain. This shape of workout additionally encourages the frame to offer feel-properly hormones known as endorphins that act as herbal painkillers.

Helps reduce stress

Engaging in yoga requires focusing for your breathing, motion, and how your body works to perform the interest. This creates a moving meditation that allows lessen stress, promotes relaxation, and improves intellectual clarity. Like meditation, yoga enables promote a first rate temper, relieves anxiety and depression, and is tremendous for reinforcing yourself guarantee.

As referred to above, any exercise that permits the body produce revel in-appropriate hormones that act as natural pressure relievers is first rate for alleviating pressure.

It enables decorate flexibility

Chair yoga calls for you to transport and bend in lots of processes. Flexibility is of most importance due to the fact the carrying activities or poses accompanied contain bending, twisting, and loose motion. And in spite of the reality that the dearth of flexibleness typically occurs due to antique age, the reality is which you need to exercise if you need to maintain your flexibility.

That is why chair yoga is crucial: it demanding situations your body to boom your shape of motion and decorate your mobility. The physical games worried are very beneficial for enhancing the ability of humans the least bit levels and a long time. The greater you have were given interplay inside the ones chair yoga sports/poses, the greater flexible you emerge as.

Chapter 2: Warm-Ups

Warming up may be very vital with regards to any bodily interest. It could be very essential because it enables save you accidents and enhances your body's regular performance. When you warmness-up, blood drift for your muscle mass increases thru as an entire lot as 75%.

There is a way of life in yoga in that you want first of all advantageous warmness-ups, often called vinyasa flows. The term vinyasa is frequently used to mean hyperlink breathing to motion. Most of the fine and comfy-up wearing occasions are usually very short and could extraordinary take in approximately 10 minutes of it slow.

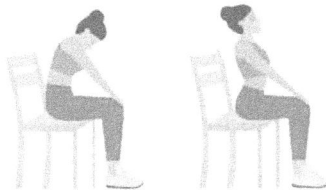

Here are some of the fast and smooth warmth-up bodily video games on the way to strive:

Cat-Cow Pose

This clean pose is terrific for stretching and shifting the joints of your backbone and hips. The warmness-up workout calls with a view to take a seat down down in a snug chair and feature.

Here is a way to pass about it.

1.   Begin through using sitting at an attitude of ninety degrees along side your once more without delay and coping with in advance.

2.   Place your fingers on your knees and take a deep breath.

three. Now slowly arch your back inwards until you're right now going via upwards as masses as you could.

4. Remain in that function for five to 10 seconds in advance than going lower back to your actual characteristic.

five. Repeat the equal approach approximately ten times till you sense your backbone and hips are properly stretched.

The Lotus Pose

One of the pleasant and quality poses you could get into is the seated lotus pose. The purpose of this exercise is to assist settle your thoughts as you open up your frame to the alternative bodily video games and own you're about to have interaction in.

Actually, maximum human beings propose beginning with this method earlier than undertaking any exercising— in case you meditate regularly, you might be extra aware of this pose.

This is the manner you do it.

1. Start with the useful resource of making sure you're seated in a pleasant and

comfortable function. You can add some cushions or a blanket in your seat.

2.   If possible, try to move your legs in the the front of every specific. Make certain to pass them as a whole lot as you could. You can use your fingers to push them as loads as you can. However, be careful no longer to pressure yourself.

three. Place your arms for your knees and lightly rock from side to side on the same time as permitting your pelvis to tilt gently. As you go with the flow, try to find a place in which your torso feels greater natural.

4.   Slowly breathe inside and outside till you enjoy your body is snug and your muscle organizations spread out to extra bodily games.

Arms Upward Pose

The palms overhead pose is any other high-quality and clean warmth-up workout that permits you to attempt. The fundamental concept within the lower back of this warmness-up recurring is to assist stretch and improve your top frame additives, which encompass your again, hands, and shoulders. You can without problem do this pose in a seated or reputation function.

Here is the manner you pass about it.

1.	The first step is to make sure you're seated in a snug characteristic along facet your back right away and going thru forward.

2.	Take a deep breath and slowly convey each your palms in advance till they'll be perpendicular to your chest.

3.	Now slowly sweep your hands up while however stretched all the way out until they'll be without delay and above your head.

4.	Remain in that role for about 10 to twenty seconds earlier than returning your palms to their true position.

5.	Repeat the equal manner about 20 instances without bringing your palms to their resting feature.

Boat Pose

This is a extra superior however beneficial form of heat-up workout that is awesome for stretching your middle muscle organizations (stomach and returned muscle agencies) and your the front leg muscle businesses. The pose is proper for beginners who've by no means completed yoga earlier than and people who're out of form. If you've got were given lower back troubles, this is a first-rate way to warmth up.

Here is a way to do it.

1.   Start with the useful resource of sitting at the floor along side your knees barely bent and toes right now at the ground. Place your arms at the floor honestly along your hips.

2.   Now gently carry your palms approximately a foot —or so— within the once more of you on the same time as you bend your elbows a piece backward to offer sufficient assist to hold your weight.

three. Slowly deliver your ankles collectively while maintaining your legs immediately. Raise them from the ground slowly till you lean on your torso approximately 30 to 45 stages.

4.   Remain in that function for about 20 seconds earlier than returning in your proper feature.

5.   Repeat the identical way about 20 instances on the equal time as maintaining a regular breath.

Sitting Twists

The sitting twists motion is a high-quality warmness-up recurring that let you benefit a few rotational moves into your backbone to assist beautify your flexibility, power, and movement. You can with out problems do the habitual either whilst repute or sitting down.

Here is a way to move about doing the exercise.

1.   Start with the aid of sitting down in a snug function collectively along with your legs carefully crossed within the front of you.

2.   Now slowly twist your higher frame inside the course of the proper until you're absolutely dealing with to your proper however together with your in the again of certainly rooted down. Remain in that role for about 10 seconds.

3.   Slowly pass in your unique characteristic earlier than twisting to your left facet and posing in that role for approximately 10 seconds.

4.   Ensure which you twist your higher body detail as masses as viable however with out straining your self an excessive amount of.

Upward Plank Pose

Like the traditional plank pose, the upward plank pose is a version of the conventional exercising ordinary this is super for warming up your center and leg muscle groups.

It is likewise first-rate for taking off your chest, which permits ease your ability to engage in and carry out unique wearing sports which includes standing poses and more. This is a greater superior form of warm-up exercise, but each person, even beginners, can control to do it.

Here is the way to cross approximately it.

1.   Start via sitting down quite in truth along with your legs stretched without delay earlier than you.

2.   Now region your hands beside your hips before slowly taking them approximately an inch within the returned of your back at the side of your elbows slightly bent.

three. Make certain your arms are robust enough to keep your weight earlier than lifting your torso slowly from the floor all of the manner up as an awful lot as feasible.

4.   Remain in that function for about 20 seconds in advance than returning on your unique feature. Repeat this method

approximately 20 instances till you feel your center and leg muscle groups have end up unfastened sufficient.

Leaning Forward Pose

The leaning beforehand pose warms up your center and leg muscle groups and is remarkable for enhancing flexibility and mobility for your hips and spinal joints to help relieve any stiffness. It might be a bit more strenuous than one-of-a-kind heat-up carrying activities, however it's far high-quality for getting you warmed up in advance than you start jogging out.

Here is the manner you move about doing the exercising.

1.   Start via sitting in the lotus position of your desire. Consider putting a blanket or a pillow beneath for maximum comfort.

2.   Now increase your shin within the the front of the opportunity and come into the pose, as illustrated within the image. Make positive not to pressure too much.

three. Push your palms as a protracted way as possible till you experience a moderate anxiety for your once more muscle groups. Stay in that feature for approximately 20 seconds earlier than happening your precise role.

4.   Repeat the same method numerous times until your middle muscular tissues and decrease returned experience properly stretched.

Seated Shoulder Rolls

This is but every different clean warm temperature-up routine that allows release the anxiety to your shoulder blades and pinnacle arm muscle. The exercise everyday is easy sufficient for anybody to do, and it's far extremely good to help open up your muscle tissues in advance than beginning your exercising.

Here is the way you go approximately doing the exercising.

1.   Start via sitting down resultseasily, together with your again without delay and legs at a 90-degree perspective.

2.   Place your hands to your knees or thighs and take a deep breath.

three. Slowly shrug your shoulders ahead and backward till you may draw a circle in the air with them.

4.   Continue with the moves in a clockwise movement for approximately 30 seconds, then repeat the identical in an anti-clockwise movement for every different 30 seconds.

Chapter 3: Breathing Exercises

When you enjoy worn-out or worn out from a exercise normal, most of the time, it's because of the truth your chest and frame, in current, had been no longer organized for the strain. That is why you find out your self panting uncontrollably, even in advance than you're midway via the workout. That's why it's important to put together your body for the massive or non-stop respiration as a manner to take place as you discern out.

Here are a few respiratory physical sports to help you get into the proper mind frame and open up your frame to the wearing sports you're approximately to interact in.

Square Breathing Movement

This respiratory exercise includes breathing in, respiration out, and preserving your breath. These moves are speculated to be completed inside the same amount of time.

The concept of a square is to assist make sure which you recall the breaths need to be equal. This exercise is likewise recovery and assist you to lighten up and loosen up. Here is the way you do it.

1.   Sit pretty genuinely collectively along with your decrease back immediately.

2.   Place your arms in your knees or thighs, where you enjoy most cushty.

three. Silently breathe in up to the depend variety of four before retaining your breath for some other take into account of four.

four.   Again, silently breathe out for a rely of for in advance than shielding your breath for the same quantity of time.

5.   Repeat this manner for about 30 seconds or so.

Intentional Breathing

Being on pinnacle of things of your respiration is important because it permits you avoid getting wiped out without trouble or rapid on the same time as walking out.

This respiratory technique introduced with the resource of the usage of Dutch immoderate athlete Wim Hof is amazing for enhancing ordinary performance and optimizing health in favored. The key problem with this exercise is the aim, not your frame actions.

Here is the manner you circulate about it.

1.   Make excellent to sit down in a pleasant and comfortable function.

2.   Gently area your palms to your knees or thighs —anywhere you enjoy most snug.

3.   Slowly take a deep breath, then breath out; maintain with this exercising till you shape a spherical motion.

four.   Continue the respiratory styles for about 30 to forty cycles.

5.   Once completed with the ultimate spherical, maintain your breath in for as long as you may.

Twist Breaths

This respiratory everyday is extremely good for developing blood and air circulate on your middle muscle agencies. It is outstanding for ensuring your hands and toes are warm, particularly inside the occasion that they commonly get bloodless. If you're about to exercising session inside the morning or are going to a cold location to schooling consultation, this method may be very beneficial.

Here is the way you do it.

1.   Sit collectively along with your legs stretched out and as extensive as viable.

2.   Take sluggish and shallow breathes that will help you relax and relax.

three. Slowly start to twist on your proper as you allow your fingers to transport freely.

4.   Make sure to respire in as you center and exhale as you twist.

five.   You can choose out to boost your legs from the floor as you twist to make certain you're snug.

6.   Continue alternating from left to proper till you enjoy properly stretched out.

The Skull Shining Breath

This is commonly the pass-to-workout even as you need to heat up rapid and with out problem. It is a splendid heat-up recurring that permit you to feel energized and warmth. This makes it the right warmness-up exercising at the same time as you're feeling cold or sluggish or maybe while you need to exercise consultation within the morning.

Here is the manner you skip about it.

1.   Find a pleasing and snug place to sit and loosen up.

2.   Place your palms for your thighs or knees —anywhere you experience maximum comfortable.

three. Take a few deep and shallow breathes. Make sure to respire in reality via your nose and sincerely thru your mouth.

4. Now take a deep breath and while you're three-quarters of the way via your nose, exhale sharply thru your mouth. As you exhale, try to force the air out the use of your diaphragm and abdominal muscular tissues.

five. Repeat this technique for approximately 10 to twenty cycles while looking how you breathe.

Ujjayi Breath

Ujjayi, this means that fine, denotes the truth that each inhalation and exhalation is a celebration of lifestyles. The concept of this normal is to assist make sure that you're feeling heat indoors; it furthermore maintains your thoughts focused at the prevailing 2d. It is pretty specific in that you have to experience and pay interest the entire way as you circulate. It is also called the "oceanic breath" because of the fact in case you listen cautiously to the cycles, you'll listen the sound of waves coming inner and out of the shore.

Here is the way you do it.

1.   Find a cushty role in which to sit even as managing in advance.

2.   Place your hands for your elements somewhere in your knees or thighs.

3.   Take a few breaths, then carefully rest your tongue inside the again of the the the front of your tooth.

4.   Inhale via your nose as you create a constriction within the lower back of your throat till you create a gentle wheezing sound.

5.   Try and maintain the constriction in the back of your throat to assist preserve the wheezing sound as you exhale.

6.   Once carried out exhaling, push your navel into your stomach to remove any last air.

Bellows Breathing

Unlike the other kinds of respiratory, this is an severe respiration technique that consists of a chain of effective inhalations and exhalations. This manner if you have respiration troubles or cannot address active breathing, you want to not have interaction on this exercise. Otherwise, in case you want to strengthen your float, you could strive it.

Here is a manner to head approximately it.

1.   Find a place to sit down together with your once more resting on the backrest.

2.   Place your hands to your torso and take a deep breath.

three. Now take a pointy and deep breath such that your diaphragm falls below till your lungs can't preserve any greater air.

four.   Quickly and sharply allow all of the air out as rapid as viable, the use of your diaphragm to get rid of any remnant air.

five.   Hold your breath for about 10 seconds in advance than repeating the stairs above for about 4 rounds of ten breaths.

Cooling Breaths

Another extraordinary respiration method that could display very beneficial for calming down and focusing your concept is the cooling breaths. Also referred to as Seetakari, this respiration routine is extraordinary for folks who constantly revel in heat or heat, even on a cold day.

If you'd like to without troubles and speedy chill out, then you could try this respiratory everyday. It is likewise incredible for cooling you down while you're ill or experiencing a fever or heat flushes and would love to relax.

Here is the manner you drift about it.

1.   Find a cushty vicinity to sit down down and place your hands in your knees.

2.   Close your eyes and gently take a deep breath.

three. Gently supply your better and decrease tooth together on the same time as allowing your lips to return lower back again apart.

four. Slowly and deeply thru the space on your enamel till you're making a hissing sound.

5.   Now close to your lips and expel the air thru your nose for about 10 mins and slowly increase the tempo at some point of times of five mins.

Alternate Nostril Breathing

This is one of the simplest yogic deep respiration because it is straightforward and proper now to the issue. It doesn't require an awful lot work because of the reality your hands will do the provide you with the outcomes you need. It is amazing for inducing sluggish rhythmic respiration that is exceptional for calming down, and whilst you switch the rims, it consists of every elements of your thoughts.

Here is the way you do it.

1.   Find a comfortable characteristic to take a seat in together together with your lower back right away.

2.   Using your right thumb, close to your proper nose after which place your index and middle finger among your eyebrows as your small finger dangles inside the air.

3.   Exhale absolutely using your left nostril and step by step allow the air lower decrease back in. Once the inhalation reaches its peak, rapid launch the left nostril and near your right nostril. You can now exhale through the right nostril and maintain alternating for approximately ten rounds.

Lion's Breath

This is a brilliant yogic breathing technique this is very beneficial for assuaging anxiety to your face and chest. It is also known as Simsahana or lion's pose, and it is easy to do. The breathing method is likewise exciting and soothing.

Here is the manner you do it.

1.   Find a comfortable place to sit down and relax.

2.   Place your arms to your knees or thighs, collectively along side your fingers spread out.

3.   Open your eyes huge and take a deep breath.

four.   As you do step 3, open your mouth and stick your tongue out as hundreds as you can on the identical time as ensuring to hold it as close as feasible for your chin.

five.   Now tighten your throat muscle groups and exhale thru your mouth as you are making the 'ha' sound.

6.   You can also moreover even attempt to test the pinnacle of your nose or the center of your eyebrows as you do it.

7.   Repeat the way for about 2 to 3 breaths.

Focus Breathing Technique

This is however a few other respiration technique that permits you become more focused and aware of your respiration. It usually consists of the use of terms and interest phrases. The method is extra like hypnotherapy, but the motive is to make you experience extra calm and comfortable.

To carry out this approach, you want to discover a word that makes you calm or glad. It may be any word so long as your mind can awareness on it and bring you a few experience of belonging or consciousness.

Here is the way you flow approximately performing this ordinary.

1.   Begin through sitting down in a pleasing and cushty location.

2.   Slowly recognition your thoughts in your respiration with out changing the manner you're respiration.

3.   Gradually shift out of your regular to deep respiratory, alternatively to normal

breathing. Take be aware of the actions on your stomach as you breathe.

four.   You can try placing your hand for your lower stomach to phrase the way it rises and falls as you breathe.

5.   As you breathe out, ensure you exhale all of the air out of your lungs.

6.   As you change amongst regular and deep respiratory, popularity on the phrase or word you selected to assist make certain you're snug as heaps as viable.

Chapter 4: Chair Yoga Poses For Seniors

The proper aspect with chair yoga is that there's a pose or exercise in particular proper for all body muscle tissues. It is essential to obtain every muscle for your body because it ensures which you artwork on all muscular tissues. There are also chair yoga poses that in form people of all tiers, whether you're a pro or a novice.

Here are some of the top notch chair yoga poses for seniors:

Seated Mountain Pose

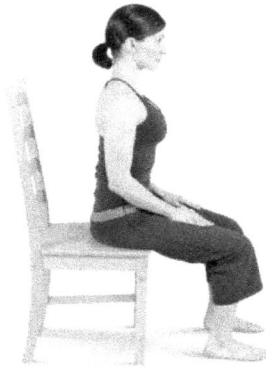

The first pose you can do is the seated mountain pose. It is mostly a very simple pose this is right for engaging your middle and focusing your breath. It is commonly the first pose you will maximum probably do each time you want to perform any chair yoga normal.

Here is the manner you do it.

1.   While sitting down, take a deep breath and prolong your backbone as a good deal as feasible.

2.   Slowly breathe out as you push your sitz bone (the bottom of your pelvis) into the chair. Make wonderful you form a ninety-degree mind-set collectively together with your thighs, decrease lower back, and legs.

three. Again, take a deep breath, then slowly exhale as you push your shoulders down and returned. Make splendid to interact your center muscle tissues and loosen up your fingers by using the usage of using your aspect.

four. Remain in that function for approximately 10 seconds as you breathe generally.

Chair Forward Bend

This yoga pose might be a tad strenuous for humans with once more problems, but it's far super for stretching your center and lower back muscle tissue. It allows you to be as flexible as viable at the same time as being as comfortable as possible, making it loads less tough. Therefore, in case you've been having lower again problems, then this chair yoga pose can help make bigger your backbone and decrease the tension in your lower again muscle groups.

Here is the manner you go with the flow approximately it:

1.   Start via sitting down effortlessly collectively along with your decrease again right now.

2.   Place your hands on your knees or thighs and take a deep breath.

3.   Bring your arms collectively earlier than your pelvic place and unfold your legs aside.

4.   Now slowly bend down at the side of your fingers in advance than you till they contact the ground between your feet.

five.   Remain in that feature for about 10 seconds earlier than going back on your particular position.

6.   Repeat the equal approach for about 20 to 30 reps.

One-Sided Arm Lifts

This chair yoga pose is excellent for strengthening your lungs, chest, and shoulders at the identical time as appealing your abs, making it a super exercising ordinary for strengthening your higher frame muscle.

The exercise recurring is probably very regarding and a piece advanced, but it's far excellent for organising up your body muscle mass. It is a version of the in advance lean pose however more effective.

Here is the manner you do it:

1.   Start through sitting down in a pleasing and snug area.

2.   Gradually bend into the ahead bend role, then take a deep breath.

3.   With your hands at the floor, slowly have interaction your chest and twist to your left as you exhale.

four.   Slowly raise your left arm as loads as viable, then appearance up at your arm.

5.   Remain in that characteristic for approximately 20 seconds as you maintain your respiration.

6.   Go decrease again on your unique role and repeat the same manner collectively with your right factor.

Seated Pigeon Pose

The seated pigeon pose is a great workout recurring that permits make more potent your groin, glutes and leg muscle organizations at the equal time as stimulating your digestive device. As the call suggests, the pose imitates a characteristic that most pigeons typically generally tend to anticipate. This newbie-pleasant pose doesn't require a bargain artwork.

Here is the way you do the pose.

1.   Start via honestly sitting down with your fingers to your knees or thighs.

2.   Take a deep breath earlier than keeping your left ankles with both fingers.

three. Slowly bring your left leg sideways inside the route of your proper knee as you breathe out.

4.   Place your left ankle to relaxation for your proper thigh or knee, then stay in that feature for approximately 20 seconds.

5.   Return your leg to its particular function earlier than repeating the equal manner on the facet of your right leg.

Reverse Arm Hold

The opposite arm keep is a fantastic and easy exercising ordinary that allows open up your chest and stretch your arm muscle groups. It is also incredible for helping you loosen up and lighten up. The high-quality element approximately the pose is that it is beginner-exceptional and can be accomplished via nearly absolutely every person at any area as long as you're seated.

Here is the way you do the pose:

1.   Start thru finding a cushty area to take a seat down down whilst making sure your once more is immediately.

2.   Take a deep breath, then stretch every your hands with the aid of your thing as an entire lot as feasible.

3.   Bring every your palms all over again, then bend them at your elbow such that your right arm can touch your left elbow and vice versa.

4.   Slowly clasp your hands collectively and gently add some resistance via pulling your fingers upwards.

five.   Remain in that position for about 20 seconds in advance than returning on your original role.

Arm Spiral Pose

The arm spiral pose is a amateur-amazing chair yoga exercising everyday this is incredible for organising up your shoulders, stretching your palms, and improving the motion for your body. At a glance, you may think that the pose is only a waste of time and energy, however it is pretty effective in case you do it the proper way.

Here is the way you pass about doing the pose:

1.   Start through sitting down in a nice, snug location at the side of your once more right away.

2.   Take a deep breath, then convey every your hands forwards.

three. Carefully wrap every your hands spherical every other as masses as you can till you shape a spiral.

4.   Slowly try to grab your shoulders with contrary palms as if you're hugging yourself.

five. Lift your elbows and live in that characteristic for approximately 20 seconds.

6.   Go again for your specific role in advance than doing the pose anti-clockwise.

Seated Star Pose

The seated famous individual pose is one amazing exercise recurring that entails maximum of the muscular tissues to your frame. It is exceptional for lengthening, strengthening, and aligning your backbone and body. It is also novice-pleasant and can be completed through the use of pretty a great deal each person.

Here is the manner you bypass approximately it:

1.	Start by means of manner of sitting down in a pleasing snug area alongside facet your lower lower returned instantly

2.	Place your palms for your knees or thighs, then take a deep breath.

3.	Slowly extend your palms for your aspect as a great deal as possible, then carry them.

4.	Now step by step unfold your legs extensive and lift them as a lot as you could as nicely.

5.	Hold your breath for 2 mins and stay in that function for 2 mins as properly.

6.	Go back on your precise position, then repeat the technique for ten to 20 reps.

Seated Warrior

If you're seeking out a greater advanced shape of chair yoga, then the seated warrior is extremely good for you. Even although it is pretty related to, it's miles very useful because it allows provide a boost to your center muscle groups, glutes, and leg muscle groups. It is also very beneficial in improving circulation to your frame.

Here is the way you do it.

1. Start with the beneficial aid of sitting down in a nice and cushty vicinity. Consider placing a pillow or a blanket for this pose.

2. Take a deep breath and slowly twist in your right such that your right leg is at the right aspect of the seat and your left leg is stretched immediately behind you.

three. Bring your fingers easy, then exhale slowly as you boom them proper now into the air.

four. Remain in that function for about 20 seconds earlier than returning for your specific function.

five. Repeat the same approach with the opportunity aspect.

One Leg Stretch

The One Leg Stretch pose is outstanding for stretching and lengthening your backbone and leg muscle tissues. It is form of just like the ahead bend lean pose however slightly exceptional. It is probably a bit strenuous for you or humans with again issues, but it's far splendid for boosting your frame's skip. The pose is quite clean to do in case you set up enough try or push your self —don't overdo it.

Here is the way you pass about doing this chair yoga pose:

1.   Begin with the resource of sitting down with no trouble collectively along with your decrease again right now and your hands on your knees or thighs.

2.   Take a deep breath, then slowly supply your left leg in advance.

three. While preserving the proper leg bent, lean down slowly till you may contact your left leg toes collectively with your left hand.

four. Stretch as lots as feasible, then stay in that characteristic for approximately 20 seconds before returning to your authentic feature.

five. Repeat the same method at the side of your exceptional side, then don't forget to exhale without a doubt as you bypass lower back on your original position.

6. Do this manner for approximately 20 to 30 reps.

Shoulder Circle Rolls

This exercising strengthens your better again muscular tissues and improves flexibility in the shoulder blades. It is pretty easy and amateur-wonderful however super for boosting circulate and relieving your arm muscle tissues of any anxiety construct-up. It is truely beneficial to try this exercise in advance on for your exercise ordinary.

Here is the way you do it.

1.   Sit without a trouble in a pleasant and comfortable seat collectively along side your lower again without delay and going via in advance.

2.   Take a deep breath, then vicinity the pointers of your fingers on top of your shoulders.

three. Slowly increase your shoulders up and beforehand, then immediately deliver them down and backward until you shape circles collectively with your shoulders.

Chapter 5: Chair Neck Rolls

The neck muscle businesses are commonly unnoticed in maximum exercise exercises, but maximum people forget about approximately that neck muscular tissues are very crucial.

They are alleged to be constantly stretched to assist prevent stiff necks, that are normally very painful and uncomfortable. It additionally permits ensure that your backbone is properly aligned, with proper flow into taking place to your head. This technique can also moreover appear clean, but it is able to artwork wonders to your nervous gadget whilst you consist of respiratory techniques.

Here is a way to do yoga neck rolls.

1.   Begin through sitting down effortlessly collectively with your lower again without delay and handling in advance.

2.   Take a deep breath, then take your neck upwards and backward as an entire lot

as you can, then exhale as you deliver your neck all the way down to your chin.

three. Continue with the lower back and in advance actions for about 20 seconds on the identical time as ensuring to stretch your neck muscle agencies as plenty as you can.

4.	Once you move once more for your true function, shift your neck within the direction of your left such that your left ear is touching your left shoulder. Remain in that role for approximately 10 seconds in advance than going decrease decrease again for your authentic feature.

five.	Repeat the equal technique with your right detail but make certain to utilize respiratory strategies as you do so.

6.	Once finished with steps 4 and five, slowly tilt your face to the right as masses as feasible earlier than tilting your face over again to the left as a fantastic deal as possible.

7.   Continue with the actions for about 20 seconds earlier than tilting your head in a round movement as you wind up.

Supported Forward Bend Pose

For this pose, you'll need to have seats or a place to region your legs on the same time as doing it. It is a variation of the beforehand lean bend, but it is more demanding and effective at improving flexibility and releasing anxiety. This workout is likewise great for aligning your backbone and strengthening your leg muscle corporations.

Here is the manner you pass approximately doing it.

1.   Start with the aid of way of setting seats managing each different and close to collectively.

2.   Sit down in one of the chairs and location your legs on the opposite chair in the front of you.

3.   Make high-quality you're cushty, then take a deep breath before leaning ahead till you could touch your toes collectively together with your fingertips.

4.   Go as low as feasible; if you may touch your ankles, the higher.

five.   Remain in that role for approximately 30 seconds in advance than returning for your precise characteristic.

6.   Continue with the movements for approximately 20 reps till your back muscle tissue are well stretched.

Seated Half-Forward On Toes Pose

If you'd want to make your chair yoga exercising recurring extra thrilling, that is the pose for you. This is each other version of the ahead lean bend pose, however it's miles a tad much less hard to do. The pose is incredible for strengthening arm muscle groups, hips, center muscle tissues, and feet. It is also first rate for improving motion inside the body.

Here is the way you move about doing the pose.

1.   Start by using way of sitting down in a pleasant and comfortable vicinity.

2.   Take a deep breath, then deliver both your hands beforehand.

three. Slowly bring them up as you breathe out as a whole lot as feasible, then lean in advance a piece.

four. Raise your feet such which you're helping yourself together with your toes and remain in that feature for approximately 20 seconds.

5.   You can try to bend your elbows to form 90 levels collectively collectively with your palms.

Hand Clenches

This smooth chair yoga pose is outstanding for buying equipped your frame for an intense exercise or growing blood motion on your fingers. It is also super for strengthening your arms and shoulder muscle tissue even as enhancing flexibility. Hand clenches are newbie-extraordinary and can be accomplished quite a good deal everywhere so long as you're seated without difficulty.

Here is the way you do it.

1. Start thru sitting down in a nice, cushty area together together together with your another time right now and handling ahead.

2. Take a deep breath, then slowly boost your hands in advance as at once as possible.

3. Exhale, then open up your arms through spreading out your hands.

4. While although in that function, make a fist on each arms, then release; make a fist over again, then launch. Make fine to clench your fist as an lousy lot as viable and hold your hands right now and perpendicular, don't lower them!

5. Continue developing a fist and freeing it till you sense no tension in your palms.

Cactus Raised Arms Pose

This is a wonderful startup exercise regular that improves your motion and versatility, getting ready you for more immoderate exercise sporting activities. The cactus raised arms pose is remarkable for strengthening your palms, shoulders, and chest muscle groups. It is likewise novice-extremely good and can be performed via pretty much definitely all of us.

Here is the way to move approximately doing this chair yoga pose.

1.   Start with the aid of sitting down in a pleasant, comfortable function whilst going through ahead.

2.   Inhale, and on the equal time as retaining your backbone immediately, enlarge your fingers big and push your chest outwards.

three. Once you increase your hands without delay beside you, bend your elbows and lift your hands to form ninety stages collectively along with your palms.

four.   Remain in that function for 20 to 30 seconds earlier than returning on your precise position.

five.   Repeat the identical manner for approximately 20 reps.

Goddess Pose

This is a great novice-pleasant exercise routine that enables decorate motion and versatility. It additionally lets in strengthen the hips, knees, and pelvic muscle groups.

Here is the way you do it.

1.   Start by using the usage of sitting down conveniently however as opposed to going via in advance, sit down down at the same time as managing backward.

2.   Spread your legs as huge as feasible alongside side your ft declaring.

three. Hold the backrest for help, then inhale and exhale generally.

four.   Hold that feature for about 20 seconds before loosening your legs and stretching them in advance.

five.   If you're up for a project, you could keep off right into a squat in the back of the chair and hold right away to it for assist.

6.   Remember to maintain your respiratory regular as you perform the exercise habitual.

Half-Moon Pose

Unlike the alternative chair yoga poses, this one calls for you to face on your ft; but, you'll nevertheless rely on the chair for assist. This workout ordinary is tremendous for strengthening many muscular tissues in your frame, which incorporates the chest, hamstrings, better decrease lower back and shoulders, center and arm muscle mass. The pose is likewise great for reinforcing flow into and flexibility.

Here is the way you bypass about doing the exercising.

1.   Start with the useful resource of repute right now in the the front of the seat.

2.   Inhale, then slowly lower your frame until you contact the seat with your fingers. Go decrease over again until you vicinity your forearm at the seat.

three. Use your proper hand for useful useful resource, then enhance your left hand.

four.   Slowly decorate your left leg till it's far perpendicular to your frame. Ensure you're balanced, together along with your right forearm is imparting sufficient help.

5.   Remain in that position for about 20 seconds in advance than returning to your proper feature.

6.   Repeat the identical approach together together with your left component.

Chair Sit-Ups

Sit-usaare a commonplace workout ordinary for max humans. They have validated to be very powerful, and people chair sit down-united statesare no exception. They help enhance your electricity and improve your center muscle companies, in particular your abs. Chair sit down-united statesare splendid for boosting flow and starting your frame for an severe exercising. The nice distinction among this and the normal sit down down-u.S.A.Most people recognize is that for this, you'll need a chair.

Here is the way you do it.

1.   Place a chair in the the front of you, then lie down whilst going via forward.

2.   Bring your legs up and place them at the seat. Move as close to as possible to the seat such that your legs form ninety levels.

3.   With your palms beside you, take a deep breath and exhale, then slowly supply them in the back of your head.

4.   Interlock your arms in advance than taking a deep breath. Slowly beautify your head as heaps as possible with the cause of reaching your thighs or knees along with your forehead.

5.   Once you acquire to your thighs or knees as a extraordinary deal as feasible, move decrease back to laying down flat and exhale.

6.   Repeat the same technique for about twenty reps. You can attempt alternating from left to proper as you do the take a seat-ups.

Reverse Warrior Pose

This is another model of the normal warrior pose, however it's far extra regarding and strenuous. This chair yoga pose is outstanding for strengthening almost all the muscle businesses for your body, which consist of the neck, higher once more, hamstrings, chest, knees, and hips. It is also awesome for enhancing flexibility and drift in your body.

Here is the manner you move approximately doing the workout.

1.   Start with the useful resource of sitting down in a pleasing and comfortable feature; keep in mind setting a pillow or a cushion at the seat.

2.   Take a deep breath, then slowly shift your proper leg to the proper aspect of your seat to form ninety levels, then stretch your left leg inside the back of you.

three. Exhale, then shift your top frame to face your proper side.

four. Once you input into the warrior characteristic, shift your decrease once more backward till you could touch your left leg together together with your left arm, then growth your right hand in the air.

five.   See the photo above for a more correct instance of what to do.

Crescent High Lunge Twists

The crescent high lunge twists are excellent for strengthening the hips, gluteus, higher decrease back, shoulders, and arms. This exercise ordinary is likewise brilliant for boosting flow into and versatility of your joints, and it permits stretch the muscle groups on your body. The exercise habitual is a bit greater strenuous than maximum different chair yoga poses, but it's far pretty effective and useful. It is a version of the thing chair twists but extra advanced.

Here is a way to transport about it.

1.   Start by means of sitting down and not the use of a hassle collectively along with your face beforehand.

2.   Take a deep breath, then deliver your right leg to the proper thing of your seat and stretch your left leg within the again of you to the left of the chair.

Chapter 6: Bolster Head Arms Pose

This is a newbie-pleasant workout normal that facilitates assist the palms and shoulders, hips out of doors, lower back and knees. It is likewise a totally comfortable chair yoga pose that lets in enhance flexibility, stability, and circulate for your frame. This chair yoga pose is a variation of the praying Buddha pose, but you may need a chair as a way to act because of the fact the assist machine.

Here is how you may pass about doing it.

1.   Start by way of the use of sitting down close to a chair handling you.

2.   Place a pillow or a blanket underneath then you definitely clearly move your legs as tested within the photograph underneath.

three. Place each your arms on the seat and fold them.

four.   Slowly lean ahead and relaxation your head at the back of your fingers.

5. Stay in that feature for approximately 20 seconds earlier than goings lower decrease lower back to your unique position.

6. Make fine to inhale and exhale at a few level inside the complete approach.

Downward Facing Plank Pose

The Downward Facing Plank pose is a model of the well-known plank pose. It is a sophisticated form of exercise habitual that facilitates beautify muscle corporations in your frame, together with the gluteus, hips, and psoas. It is a totally newbie-friendly exercising ordinary and is extraordinary applicable for those who can not do the ordinary plank.

Here is the way you do the pose.

1. Start with the beneficial aid of fame up right now at the back of a chair, with the backrest going thru you.

2.   Make positive you're a few inches from the chair and hold the backrest with each hands.

three. Lower your top frame difficulty as low as you may until you're going via the ground and forming 90 tiers with the chair.

four. With the help of the chair, increase your frame as a splendid deal as you may until you shape a diagonal and stand in your toes.

five.   Remain in that feature for about 20 seconds earlier than returning in your real feature.

6.   Repeat the identical approach for approximately 20 reps.

Chair Gate Pose

The chair gate pose is a version of the sideways pose we noted in advance, however the pose is extra strenuous and powerful. It is a newbie-satisfactory exercise regular that permits assist the center, arm, and leg muscular tissues while also assisting beautify flexibility and stability.

Here is the way you do the pose.

1.   Begin with the beneficial resource of sitting down without trouble with your face in advance.

2.   Place your fingers to your thighs or your knees and take a deep breath.

three. Slowly enlarge your left leg out as a fantastic deal as you could.

four.   Gradually twist your top body sideways till you can contact your left leg along with your left hand as you stretch your proper arm upwards.

5.   Remain in that role for approximately 20 seconds earlier than returning in your true characteristic.

6.   Repeat the identical system collectively along side your proper aspect and keep alternating for ten reps.

Standing Forward Fold Pose

This is the right pose in case you'd need to make your exercise everyday a chunk greater difficult. It is probably a bit strenuous, however it's miles quite powerful in strengthening your muscular tissues, improving flexibility, and enhancing balance. Some of the muscle groups it allows to reinforce are the abs, palms and shoulders, neck, hip externals, and once more muscle groups.

Here is the way you skip approximately doing this chair yoga pose.

1.   Start thru standing in the the the front of the chair you propose to apply.

2.   Slowly raise your left leg and place it on the seat, then turn and face your right side.

three. Take a deep breath, then lower your better body as hundreds as you can until you can use your proper arm to touch your proper foot.

4.   Place your left arm on the seat to help enhance your balance and posture.

5.   Remain in that function for about 20 seconds earlier than returning to your true function.

6.   Repeat the same procedure collectively along with your distinct side.

Seated Wind Release Pose

This is some other amateur-pleasant chair yoga workout that allows provide a boost in your muscle agencies and opens up your frame in education for the workout. Some of the muscle organizations targeted by way of using this pose consist of the legs, gluteus, back, and arm muscle groups. It is quite clean to do and may be executed via pretty an lousy lot surely every person from the consolation in their seat. It is likewise exceptional for boosting flexibility and drift to your lower body muscle groups.

Here is the manner you skip about doing the exercising.

1. Start thru sitting down in a pleasing, snug location, collectively with your again directly and going through ahead.

2. Take a deep breath, then cautiously boom every your legs up as lots as you can. Make positive to hold your another time right away.

three. Wrap your hands round your legs for guide, then stay in that feature for about 20 seconds.

four. Exhale and skip over again to your authentic characteristic. Repeat the same device for about 15 reps.

5. There are variations to this pose in which you can trade elevating one leg after the opportunity. You can repeat the same way however in place of elevating each legs, enhance one leg after the possibility on the equal time as using each your hands for manual.

6. Remember to breathe normally and live in that feature for about 20 seconds in

advance than alternating with the possibility leg.

Camel Pose With Chair

There are numerous variations of this pose, however the one in focus proper proper here is the camel chair pose. This is a completely easy however powerful yoga pose that is superb for enhancing flexibility and flow into on your frame.

The camel pose with chair pose is outstanding for strengthening a massive form of muscle agencies within the body, collectively with the over again, hips, hands, and middle muscle companies. It is the lots much less strenuous form of the ordinary camel pose that calls at the manner to pass all of the manner right down to your feet.

Here is the manner you pass approximately doing the pose.

1.   Begin by using manner of way of fame close to a chair however together with your again managing it. Make certain to face a few

inches from the chair to offer sufficient room to your legs whilst you kneel.

2.   Carefully kneel and bring your fingers backward such that they'll be able to maintain the seat in the back of you.

3.   Now slowly lean lower back as an entire lot as you may till you face upwards. Make sure to hold your toes collectively and in between the chair.

four. Remain in that feature for approximately 20 seconds earlier than returning on your right position. Repeat this approach for ten reps at the identical time as ensuring you bend backward as plenty as viable.

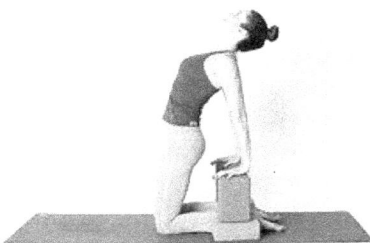

Supported Chair Camel Pose

The supported chair camel pose is a version of the camel pose we stated earlier, however this pose is much less tough in assessment. It is a beginner-first-rate exercise normal that permits enhance flexibility and strengthens the chest, fingers and shoulders, neck and knee muscle tissue. The pose is likewise remarkable for enhancing flow into on your frame and making prepared you for a exercising.

Here is the manner you bypass approximately doing the pose.

1.   Start via popularity next to a chair, together along with your lower lower back dealing with the chair and a few inches from the chair.

2.   Carefully supply your palms backward and decrease your right hand until it reaches the seat, then right away decrease your distinct arm to attain the seat.

three. Make nice to transport as lower as feasible then stay in that role for about 20 seconds in advance than going once more on your real feature

4.   Make sure to keep your respiratory everyday and hold with the device for approximately ten reps.

The Forward Bend Pose

If you've been having trouble along with your yet again muscle tissues, then this pose will flow a long way in remedying that. The ahead bend pose is high-quality for boosting flexibility and strengthening the hips, lower all over again, and center muscle tissues. It is novice-fine and may be finished by means of the usage of quite masses all of us. The pose is a model of the in advance lean pose, but in choice to being seated in the route of the workout, you stay reputation.

Here is the way you pass approximately doing the pose.

1.   Start through popularity in the front of a chair dealing with it, on the side of your lower back right now.

2.   Take a deep breath, slowly decrease your top body as low as feasible, and vicinity your arms on the seat.

three. Once you pass your hands at the chair within the the front of you, lay your head on your fingers and continue to be in that function.

4.   Make positive you preserve your legs right now: don't bend your knees.

five. Stay in that characteristic for 20 seconds in advance than returning to your precise role. Repeat the identical manner for about 20 reps till you enjoy the tension launched out of your lower again.

Standing Leg Lifts

The reputation leg lifts chair pose is a version of the regular leg lifts, however way to the chair, the manner becomes less difficult. This pose is high-quality for commencing your body for a exercising consultation, making this pose ideal as a pre-exercise ordinary.

It is also top notch for enhancing flexibility and permits red meat up muscle groups to your frame, in conjunction with the gluteus, hip, and calf muscle tissues. It is pretty easy and beginner-first-class so people of all stages can do it.

Here is the way you go approximately doing the pose.

1.   Start with the aid of using the usage of reputation in the front of a chair with its decrease again resting handling you.

2.   Place your left arm atop the backrest, then take a deep breath.

three. Slowly as you exhale, increase your proper leg and produce your proper hand again to maintain the leg at your feet.

4.   Make positive to reinforce your right leg as masses as possible and preserve your left leg proper now.

five. Remain in that position for approximately 20 seconds in advance than repeating the identical system together together with your exceptional side.

6.   Continue with the same system for approximately ten reps.

Standing Leg Stretch Chair Pose

The repute leg stretch pose is some other wonderful way to stretch and make more potent your glutes, hips, and decrease decrease lower back muscle groups. This chair yoga pose is novice-high-quality and lets in beautify flexibility to your lower body.

Here is the way you pass approximately doing the pose.

1.   Begin by means of way of status within the front of the chair collectively with your lower lower back right away.

2.   Now carefully lift your left leg and place it on the seat on the identical time as preserving it as instantly as possible. Also, make certain your right leg is right now: do no longer bend your knee.

3.   Bring your hands backward and pass them in the again of you, then lower your head down till your brow touches your knees.

four.   Remain in that characteristic for about 20 seconds in advance than repeating the equal technique along aspect your one in all a kind leg.

5.   Continue with the identical manner for ten reps.

Triangle Pose

This is a beginner-friendly chair yoga pose this is top notch for enhancing flexibility and strengthening your center, leg, and hands muscles. It is also high-quality for improving motion and stretching your body in readiness for the exercise consultation earlier.

Here is the way you do the pose.

1.   Begin through setting the chair in front of you with the backrest going through you.

2.   Slowly breathe in and location your left hand on pinnacle of the backrest.

three. Spread your legs as big as feasible, then twist your higher frame sideways toward your right as masses as feasible.

4.   Remain in that role for 20 seconds earlier than returning for your real function.

five.   Repeat the same way collectively collectively with your other facet and keep alternating for ten reps.

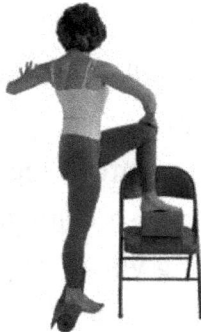

Standing Side Twists

This version of the seated factor twists permits enhance and stretch the decrease again muscle agencies, center muscular tissues, gluteus, and arm muscle mass. The repute issue twists are beginner-pleasant and perfectly suited for seniors, in particular due to the manual chair. It is also superb because of the truth, in evaluation to the seated aspect twists, the reputation component twists will will let you interact your lower stomach.

Here is the manner you move about doing the exercise.

1. Begin by way of the usage of status in front of a chair this is managing you. Ensure your returned is straight away and that you're going thru ahead before raising your left leg and putting it in your seat.

2. Place your left hand to your waist, then slowly twist towards your left as tons as you

could, then stay in that position for 10 seconds.

three. Now repeat the same method at the side of your proper element and pause for 10 seconds.

4.   Change over in your right leg, then repeat the equal process for approximately 10 reps.

five.   Continue alternating from one leg to every other for about 20 seconds.

Garland Hands-On Chair Pose

This interesting but smooth chair yoga pose is exceptional for strengthening and enhancing flexibility to your decrease stomach muscle agencies. Some of the muscle tissues impacted by using manner of this exercising consist of the gluteus, middle, hips, legs, and reduce lower back muscle mass.

Thanks to the guide provided through the chair, the chair yoga pose is pretty easy and novice-friendly. Unless you have were given a trouble collectively in conjunction with your legs, you want to with out issue do the pose.

Here is the way you circulate about doing the garland chair pose.

1.   Start through setting a seat right in front of you, then stand directly going via it.

2.   Take a deep breath, then slowly lower your body down into a squat.

3.   Breath out as you accomplish that, then vicinity each arms at the seat of the chair.

four.   Remain in that feature for about 20 seconds in advance than returning to your particular role.

5.   You also can don't forget pulling one leg out as you squat to make the exercising

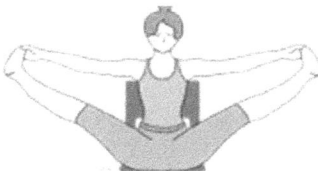

more difficult

Upward Seated Straddle

The upward seated straddle is a variation of the seated straddle we stated earlier. However, the distinction amongst the ones yoga poses is that the upwards one calls for you to be on a seat, collectively along with your legs up in the air.

This chair yoga pose is super for strengthening and stretching your leg muscle tissue, arm muscle groups, gluteus muscle groups, and decrease decrease lower back muscle groups. It is novice-friendly and amusing to engage in.

Chapter 7: Gentle Warm-Up Exercises

Neck and Shoulder Rolls in Chair Yoga

Neck and shoulder rolls are simple however effective bodily video games in chair yoga which can assist launch anxiety, lessen stiffness, and beautify flexibility within the better body. These slight moves are in particular beneficial for folks that spend lengthy hours sitting at a desk, running on a pc, or wearing strain of their neck and shoulders. Here's how to perform neck and shoulder rolls in chair yoga:

Preparation:

Sit effects on a strong chair together with your feet flat at the floor, hip-width apart.

Place your palms in your thighs or knees, arms handling down, in a comfortable and open posture.

Make remarkable your shoulders are snug and your spine is straight away.

Neck Rolls:

Step 1: Tilt Your Head Forward

Inhale deeply as you growth your chin barely.

Exhale slowly and gently, lowering your chin closer to your chest. Keep the motion easy and managed.

The again of your neck must experience clearly stretched.

Step 2: Roll Your Head to the Right

Inhale as you slowly roll your head to the right, bringing your proper ear within the course of your proper shoulder.

Exhale as you maintain the spherical motion, rolling your head down and beforehand, bringing your chin decrease decrease returned for your chest.

Feel a strain on your neck's left thing.

Inhale once more as you roll your head to the left, bringing your left ear inside the direction of your left shoulder.

Exhale as you complete the circle, returning your chin on your chest.

Step 3: Complete the Rotation

Continue the rotation for numerous breath cycles, allowing your neck to loosen up and your muscles to release anxiety.

Make the motion sluggish and conscious, being attentive to any areas of tightness.

You can carry out 3-5 rotations in a unmarried route in advance than reversing the path.

Shoulder Rolls:

Step 1: Lift Your Shoulders

Inhale deeply as you raise each shoulders closer to your ears. Feel the tension for your neck and shoulders.

Hold this role for a second, taking a deep breath.

Step 2: Roll Your Shoulders Back

Exhale as you roll your shoulders lower again and down in a round motion. Imagine drawing a circle together along with your shoulder blades.

Feel your shoulder blades moving resultseasily and releasing anxiety on your top decrease returned and neck.

Step 3: Complete the Rotation

Continue the circular movement for numerous breath cycles, allowing your shoulders to lighten up and launch any constructed-up tension.

After a few rotations, opposite the direction via manner of rolling your shoulders in advance for the equal sort of cycles.

Tips:

Maintain gradual and controlled actions in some unspecified time inside the future of each sports activities.

Never stress your head or shoulders into positions that motive ache or ache.

Keep your breath normal and coordinated with the moves for a chilled effect.

Perform neck and shoulder rolls day by day or as needed to alleviate anxiety and maintain flexibility to your top frame.

Neck and shoulder rolls in chair yoga are tremendous for promoting relaxation and lowering stiffness in the top body. They can be finished at any time all through the day, making them a available and beneficial addition to your every day ordinary, specifically when you have a sedentary lifestyle or revel in common neck and shoulder anxiety.

Wrist and Ankle Circles in Chair Yoga

Wrist and ankle circles are clean but effective bodily activities in chair yoga that can help beautify joint mobility, reduce stiffness, and beautify skip inside the wrists and ankles. These movements are particularly beneficial for seniors and folks who spend prolonged intervals sitting or have restrained mobility of their wrists and ankles. Here's a manner to carry out wrist and ankle circles in chair yoga:

Wrist Circles:

Step 1: Sit Comfortably

Begin by using the use of sitting effects in a robust chair at the facet of your ft flat at the floor and your spine right now.

Place your fingers with the hands going via all the way down to your knees or thighs.

Step 2: Extend Your Fingers

Inhale deeply as you enlarge your arms and spread them great aside.

Make tremendous your wrists are relaxed, not flexed or stretched.

Step 3: Begin the Circles

Exhale as you begin making sluggish, mild circles collectively collectively with your wrists. Imagine tracing a small circle along with your fingertips.

Continue the spherical movement for numerous breath cycles, making the circles as smooth and controlled as feasible.

You can perform 5-10 rotations in a single course in advance than reversing the direction.

Step four: Reverse the Circles

After reversing the course, perform 5-10 rotations in the opposite path.

Maintain a cushty and everyday breath within the direction of the exercise.

Ankle Circles:

Step 1: Sit Comfortably

Sit inside the equal snug chair role as for wrist circles.

Place your fingers with the fingers going via all the manner right down to your knees or thighs.

Step 2: Lift Your Foot

Inhale deeply as you improve one foot off the floor, keeping your heel related to the ground.

Point your toes away from you to activate your ankle joint.

Step three: Begin the Circles

Exhale as you start making slow, controlled circles together together together with your lifted ankle. Imagine drawing a circle together with your ft.

Continue the round motion for severa breath cycles, feeling the stretch and mobility to your ankle.

Perform five-10 rotations in a single path earlier than reversing the path.

Step four: Reverse the Circles

After reversing the direction, carry out 5-10 rotations within the contrary direction.

Maintain a relaxed breath and switch to the alternative ankle to duplicate the exercise.

Tips:

Keep the moves slow, smooth, and managed for every wrist and ankle circles.

Perform those wearing sports activities each day or as had to beautify joint mobility and decrease stiffness.

If you revel in ache or discomfort inside the route of the physical games, reduce the variety of movement or save you if vital. If the discomfort keeps, communicate with a medical physician.

Wrist and ankle circles in chair yoga are extraordinary for preserving joint fitness and reducing the risk of stiffness, specially in case you spend extended durations in a seated feature. Incorporating the ones easy movements into your every day habitual can make contributions to higher wrist and ankle flexibility, making everyday sports activities sports greater comfortable and a laugh.

Seated Cat-Cow Stretch in Chair Yoga

The Seated Cat-Cow Stretch is a slight and effective chair yoga exercise that facilitates beautify spinal flexibility, relieve tension within the once more, and sell relaxation. This version of the traditional Cat-Cow Stretch is available for people who can also have hassle getting on the floor or pick out to exercising yoga in a chair. Here's a way to carry out the Seated Cat-Cow Stretch in chair yoga:

Preparation:

Sit efficiently on a strong chair collectively at the side of your ft flat at the floor, hip-width aside.

Place your fingers on your thighs or knees, arms going through down, in a comfortable and open posture.

Make high quality your shoulders are comfortable and your spine is straight away.

Chapter 8: Seated Asanas (Poses)

Mountain Pose (Tadasana) in Chair Yoga

Mountain Pose, referred to as Tadasana in Sanskrit, is a foundational yoga pose that paperwork the idea for masses distinct poses. In chair yoga, Mountain Pose may be tailored to a seated characteristic, permitting human beings with restricted mobility or stability issues to enjoy the grounding and alignment benefits it gives. Here's the manner to perform Mountain Pose in chair yoga:

Preparation:

Sit with out problems on a sturdy chair with your feet flat on the ground, hip-width apart.

Place your palms for your thighs or knees, fingers going thru down, in a comfortable and open posture.

Ensure your spine is without delay, and your shoulders are cushty.

Mountain Pose in a Chair:

Step 1: Find Your Foundation:

Begin thru feeling the relationship of your feet to the ground. Even despite the fact that you are sitting, receive as actual along with your ft because the roots of a robust mountain.

Spread your toes massive and press them lightly into the floor, doling out your weight gently among each toes.

Step 2: Align Your Spine

Inhale deeply as you enlarge your backbone upward. Imagine every vertebra stacking on top of the alternative, growing place among them.

Engage your middle muscle tissues slightly to assist your spine on this elongated characteristic.

Step 3: Relax Your Arms:

Let your fingers relaxation without a hassle for your thighs or knees.

Allow your shoulders to melt an extended manner from your ears.

Step 4: Lift Your Chest:

Inhale and lightly improve your chest, growing area for your coronary heart middle.

Feel your ribcage boom as you breathe deeply.

Step 5: Soften Your Gaze:

Maintain a gentle gaze, looking right away earlier or barely downward.

Imagine a detail on the horizon in which you hobby your hobby.

Step 6: Breathe Mindfully:

Close your eyes in case you're snug, or maintain them softly open.

Take slow, deep breaths internal and out, keeping your interest at the sensations for your body and your connection to the ground.

Step 7: Find Stillness:

Mountain Pose is prepared locating stillness and balance, much like a mountain.

Hold the pose for 30 seconds to a minute, or as extended as it feels comfortable and calming for you.

Tips:

Maintain a experience of grounding and balance via your ft, in spite of the fact that you are sitting. Imagine them due to the fact the stable base of your mountain.

Keep your breath ordinary and comfortable, permitting it to deepen your feel of presence and grounding.

Mountain Pose is an high-quality start line for any chair yoga workout, as it lets in you set up a strong foundation and aware awareness.

Mountain Pose in chair yoga is a exquisite manner to foster a sense of groundedness, decorate posture, and increase attention of your frame and breath. It's a flexible and available pose that may be practiced through the use of individuals of each age and abilties, supplying a 2d of stillness and mindfulness within the midst of every day lifestyles.

Seated Forward Bend (Paschimottanasana) in Chair Yoga

Seated Forward Bend, called Paschimottanasana in Sanskrit, is a traditional yoga pose that stretches the backbone, hamstrings, and decrease returned muscular tissues on the same time as selling rest and versatility. In chair yoga, Paschimottanasana may be adapted to a seated function, making it available and beneficial for human beings who've trouble sitting on the floor or have restricted mobility. Here's a way to carry out a seated beforehand bend in chair yoga:

Preparation:

Sit without issue on a strong chair together with your toes flat on the ground, hip-width aside.

Place your fingers in your thighs or knees, fingers managing down, in a snug and open posture.

Ensure your backbone is at once, and your shoulders are comfortable.

Seated Forward Bend in a Chair:

Step 1: Find Your Foundation:

Begin by way of the use of sitting effects getting ready to the chair, ensuring your toes are flat on the ground.

Imagine your sitting bones rooted firmly into the chair seat, growing balance.

Step 2: Lengthen Your Spine:

Inhale deeply as you make bigger your backbone upward. You can also experience your head's crown sloping upward.

Engage your center muscle groups barely to assist your lower lower back and preserve an elongated spine.

Step three: Inhale and Lift Your Arms:

Inhale deeply as you decorate your fingers overhead, preserving them parallel to each particular.

As you inhale, boom your chest and amplify your spine even extra.

Step four: Exhale and Fold Forward:

Exhale slowly and hinge ahead at your hips, maintaining your back immediately and your fingers extended.

Allow your fingers to acquire to your toes, shins, or the chair's legs, counting on your flexibility.

If you can not attain your feet or legs pretty definitely, absolutely vicinity your hands for your thighs or knees.

Continue to fold ahead, preserving a proper away back, and lead collectively with your coronary coronary heart.

Step five: Breathe and Relax

Take slow, deep breaths as you hold the beforehand bend function.

Focus on the sensation of stretching along your spine and the backs of your legs.

Aim to keep the pose for 20-30 seconds, or longer if it is snug for you.

Step 6: Inhale to Rise

Inhale deeply as you slowly upward push decrease again to an upright sitting function.

Reach your hands overhead all over again, and then lower them to your aspects as you come to a comfortable sitting posture.

Tips:

Keep your knees barely bent if you have tight hamstrings or decrease again problems. The purpose is to revel in a mild stretch, no longer pain.

Ensure that your movement is slow and controlled in some unspecified time in the future of the pose.

If you have got any clinical situations or obstacles, speak over together with your healthcare employer or a chair yoga instructor earlier than trying Seated Forward Bend.

Seated Forward Bend in chair yoga is a tremendous way to stretch and extend the spine, enhance flexibility inside the hamstrings, and sell relaxation. Regular workout of this pose can assist alleviate anxiety within the lower back and decorate everyday posture and properly-being, making it a treasured addition for your chair yoga habitual.

Seated Twist (Ardha Matsyendrasana) in Chair Yoga

The Seated Twist, additionally referred to as Ardha Matsyendrasana, is a beneficial yoga pose for enhancing spinal flexibility, and digestion and promoting relaxation. In chair yoga, this traditional twisting pose may be tailor-made for seated workout, making it handy and effective for people with restricted mobility or stability issues.

Here's the manner to carry out Seated Twist in chair yoga:

Preparation:

Sit with out trouble on a robust chair collectively together with your toes flat at the ground, hip-width aside.

Place your arms on your thighs or knees, palms handling down, in a snug and open posture.

Ensure your backbone is at once, and your shoulders are comfortable.

Seated Twist in a Chair:

Step 1: Find Your Foundation:

Begin through sitting simply at the chair collectively with your feet flat at the ground.

Feel the relationship of your sitting bones to the chair seat, growing balance.

Step 2: Lengthen Your Spine:

Inhale deeply as you make bigger your spine upward, carrying out the crown of your head towards the ceiling.

Engage your center muscular tissues slightly to help your lower back and hold the elongated spine.

Step 3: Inhale and Lift Your Arms:

Inhale deeply as you improve your right arm overhead, preserving it parallel to the floor.

Lift your chest and extend your spine even greater as you inhale.

Step four: Exhale and Twist to the Right:

Exhale slowly and start to curl your torso to the proper. Your left hand can gently relaxation at the out of doors of your right thigh for manual.

Keep your lower lower back right now and your middle engaged as you twist.

Turn your head to the right and look over your right shoulder, if snug.

Ensure that your shoulders stay snug and far from your ears.

Step 5: Breathe and Hold:

Take slow, deep breaths as you hold the twist, feeling the moderate stretch along your spine and the twist to your torso.

Aim to preserve the pose for 20-30 seconds, or longer if it's cushty for you.

Step 6: Inhale to Release:

Inhale deeply as you slowly pass returned to the middle, bringing your right arm returned to its initial function.

Pause and take a breath to middle your self in advance than repeating the twist at the alternative aspect.

Step 7: Repeat the Twist to the Left:

Follow the equal steps, this time twisting to the left. Inhale as you elevate your left arm, and exhale as you twist.

Remember to maintain your actions sluggish and controlled.

Tips:

If you have got restrained flexibility or mobility, you may use the armrest of the chair for resource as you twist.

Be slight at the facet of your movements and by no means force your body proper right into a position that motives pain or pain.

The Seated Twist is super for selling digestion, so it may be mainly beneficial after a meal.

If you have got were given any scientific situations or obstacles, communicate over along with your healthcare issuer or a chair yoga instructor before attempting Seated Twist.

Seated Twist in Chair yoga gives an possibility to decorate spinal mobility, launch anxiety inside the decrease lower back, and sell relaxation. By incorporating this twisting pose into your chair yoga everyday, you could decorate your ordinary flexibility, digestion, and well-being on the identical time as final seated in a comfortable and on hand role.

Seated Sun Salutation in Chair Yoga

The Seated Sun Salutation is a changed version of the conventional Sun Salutation collection, tailor-made for chair yoga. It gives a moderate and energizing way to warm temperature up the body, stretch, and boom flexibility at the same time as remaining seated. This series is specifically appropriate for individuals with constrained mobility or stability problems. Here's a manner to perform the Seated Sun Salutation in chair yoga:

Preparation:

Sit without a hassle on a robust chair together along with your toes flat on the floor, hip-width apart.

Place your palms for your thighs or knees, palms managing down, in a snug and open posture.

Ensure your spine is immediately, and your shoulders are comfortable.

Seated Sun Salutation:

Step 1: Mountain Pose (Tadasana):

Inhale deeply as you reach your fingers overhead, fingers going thru every other.

Lift your chest and lengthen your spine.

Step 2: Seated Forward Bend (Paschimottanasana):

Exhale slowly and hinge beforehand at your hips, retaining your lower back right now.

Allow your palms to advantage to your ft, shins, or the chair's legs, relying for your flexibility.

Keep your knees slightly bent if wished, and maintain the stretch for a few breaths.

Step 3: Halfway Lift (Ardha Uttanasana):

Inhale and raise your better frame midway, extending your backbone beforehand and looking beforehand.

Keep your palms in your shins or thighs for guide.

Step 4: Seated Forward Bend (Paschimottanasana):

Exhale as you come to the beforehand bend, attaining for your toes or shins.

Hold for a few breaths, retaining a proper away lower decrease back.

Step five: Mountain Pose (Tadasana):

Inhale deeply as you come to the Mountain Pose, mission your fingers overhead.

Lift your chest and extend your spine.

Step 6: Seated Twist (Ardha Matsyendrasana):

Exhale and twist your torso to the proper, putting your left hand on the outdoor of your right thigh for manual.

Look over your right shoulder by way of the use of turning your head to the right.

Hold the twist for some breaths.

Step 7: Center:

As you come in your centre, take a huge breath.

Pause and take a breath to middle yourself before twisting to the left.

Step 8: Seated Twist (Ardha Matsyendrasana):

Exhale and twist your torso to the left, setting your proper hand at the outdoor of your left thigh for assist.

Look over your proper shoulder thru turning your head to the proper.

Hold the twist for some breaths.

Step nine: Center:

As you are available your centre, take a large breath.

Pause and take a breath to middle your self.

Step 10: Mountain Pose (Tadasana):

Inhale deeply as you bought your hands overhead, hands coping with every distinctive.

Lift your chest and lengthen your spine.

Step eleven: Release:

Pull your arms right proper down to your facets as you exhale.

Sit with out a problem and lighten up for a 2d, taking a few deep breaths.

Tips:

Perform each movement slowly and mindfully, coordinating your breath with the motions.

Chapter 9: Standing Poses With Chair Support

Chair-Assisted Warrior I in Chair Yoga

Chair-Assisted Warrior I is a modified version of the conventional Warrior I pose, tailored for chair yoga. This variant allows humans with constrained mobility or stability problems to enjoy the benefits of this empowering and grounding posture. Warrior I strengthens the legs stretches the torso, and promotes a experience of stability and power. Here's the way to carry out Chair-Assisted Warrior I in chair yoga:

Preparation:

Sit quite in reality on a sturdy chair collectively along with your feet flat at the ground, hip-width apart.

Place your arms on your thighs or knees, palms handling down, in a snug and open posture.

Ensure your spine is right now, and your shoulders are comfortable.

Chair-Assisted Warrior I:

Step 1: Find Your Foundation:

Begin through sitting effortlessly on the chair with your toes flat on the floor.

Imagine your sitting bones rooted firmly into the chair seat, growing stability.

Step 2: Prepare Your Leg Position:

Start collectively together with your proper leg. Inhale deeply as you carry your proper foot off the ground.

Extend your right leg at once inside the front of you and have interaction your quadriceps (thigh muscle mass).

Step 3: Find Your Balance:

While preserving your left foot flat on the ground, pivot your right foot to the proper. Your toes need to factor barely outward.

Imagine a line connecting your proper heel to your left heel, developing a slight attitude together together together with your chair.

This is the bottom on your Chair-Assisted Warrior I.

Step four: Extend Your Arms:

Inhale deeply as you amplify your fingers overhead, reaching them up toward the ceiling.

Keep your fingers dealing with every different and your fingers spread big.

Step 5: Bend Your Left Knee:

Exhale slowly as you bend your left knee, lowering your hips in the course of the chair.

Aim to create a 90-diploma mindset on the aspect of your left knee in order that it's miles aligned without delay above your left ankle.

Keep your spine upright and your gaze ahead.

Step 6: Hold and Breathe:

Take gradual, deep breaths as you hold the Chair-Assisted Warrior I pose.

Focus on the strength and balance of your lower body and the stretch in your torso.

Step 7: Release and Switch Sides:

Inhale as you slowly straighten your left knee, returning to the begin characteristic.

Lower your arms on your aspects and area your proper foot yet again at the ground.

Take a 2d to middle your self before switching to the opportunity component.

Step eight: Repeat on the Other Side:

Perform the Chair-Assisted Warrior I pose at the left aspect with the aid of lifting your left foot and pivoting it to the left.

Bend your proper knee this time and benefit your arms overhead.

Hold the pose for an same quantity of time as you in all likelihood did at the proper element.

Step nine: Release and Return to Center:

Exhale as you decrease your hands, vicinity your left foot over again on the floor, and sit down without troubles at the chair.

Tips:

Use the chair's backrest for assist if desired, specifically if balance is difficult.

Ensure that your bent knee is aligned right away above the ankle to shield your knee joint.

Chair-Assisted Warrior I may be a quick strengthening workout or held for longer intervals to construct leg electricity and stability.

If you've got any medical situations or obstacles, talk in conjunction with your healthcare organisation or a chair yoga teacher earlier than attempting Chair-Assisted Warrior I.

Chair-Assisted Warrior I in chair yoga offers an possibility to strengthen your legs, stretch your torso, and experience a enjoy of empowerment on the same time as seated in a strong and available role. Regular exercise of this pose can enhance leg energy, posture, and a feel of groundedness, making it a precious addition in your chair yoga ordinary.

Chair-Assisted Warrior II in Chair Yoga

Chair-Assisted Warrior II is a modified version of the conventional Warrior II pose, tailored for chair yoga. This version allows human beings with restricted mobility or balance problems to revel in the advantages of this empowering and grounding posture. Warrior II strengthens the legs, opens the hips, and promotes a sense of balance and strength. Here's a way to perform Chair-Assisted Warrior II in chair yoga:

Preparation:

Sit quite sincerely on a sturdy chair collectively along with your feet flat at the ground, hip-width apart.

Place your fingers in your thighs or knees, palms coping with down, in a cushty and open posture.

Ensure your spine is right away, and your shoulders are comfortable.

Chair-Assisted Warrior II:

Step 1: Find Your Foundation:

Begin through way of sitting simply at the chair along side your feet flat at the ground.

Imagine your sitting bones rooted firmly into the chair seat, developing balance.

Step 2: Prepare Your Leg Position:

Start along with your right leg. Inhale deeply as you improve your right foot off the ground.

Extend your right leg at once in the front of you and interact your quadriceps (thigh muscle tissues).

Step three: Find Your Balance:

While keeping your left foot flat on the floor, pivot your right foot to the proper. Your toes want to element to the thing, and your proper heel ought to be aligned along with your left heel.

Imagine a line connecting your right heel in your left heel, developing a immediately line together together with your chair.

Step 4: Extend Your Arms:

Inhale deeply as you increase your hands out to the rims, parallel to the ground.

Keep your fingers going via down and your arms unfold big.

Step five: Bend Your Left Knee:

Exhale slowly as you bend your left knee, reducing your hips inside the path of the chair.

Aim to create a 90-degree angle along side your left knee in order that it's far aligned right now above your left ankle.

Keep your spine upright and your gaze forward, looking over your left fingertips.

Step 6: Hold and Breathe:

Take sluggish, deep breaths as you preserve the Chair-Assisted Warrior II pose.

Focus at the strength and balance of your lower frame and the stretch on your torso.

Step 7: Release and Switch Sides:

Inhale as you straighten your left knee, returning to the start function.

Lower your hands for your factors and area your proper foot once more on the floor.

Take a 2d to middle your self in advance than switching to the alternative side.

Step eight: Repeat at the Other Side:

Perform the Chair-Assisted Warrior II pose on the left element thru lifting your left foot and pivoting it to the left.

Bend your proper knee this time, increase your palms, and look over your proper fingertips.

Hold the pose for an same quantity of time as you possibly did on the proper issue.

Step nine: Release and Return to Center:

Exhale as you decrease your palms, location your left foot over again on the ground, and take a seat with out a trouble at the chair.

Tips:

Use the chair's backrest for manual if wanted, specially if stability is tough.

Ensure that your bent knee is aligned at once above the ankle to defend your knee joint.

Chair-Assisted Warrior II may be a short strengthening workout or held for longer periods to construct leg power and balance.

If you have got got any medical conditions or boundaries, are looking for recommendation out of your healthcare business enterprise or a chair yoga teacher earlier than trying Chair-Assisted Warrior II.

Chair-Assisted Warrior II in chair yoga gives an possibility to reinforce your legs, open your hips, and experience a experience of empowerment on the equal time as seated in a sturdy and available role. Regular exercise of this pose can enhance leg power, posture, and a feeling of groundedness, making it a valuable addition in your chair yoga routine.

Chair-Assisted Triangle Pose (Trikonasana) in Chair Yoga

Chair-Assisted Triangle Pose is a changed version of the conventional Triangle Pose (Trikonasana) tailored for chair yoga. This version permits humans with confined mobility or stability troubles to revel in the benefits of this incredible yoga pose. Triangle Pose allows stretch and make more potent the legs, open the hips, and beautify flexibility. Here's the manner to perform Chair-Assisted Triangle Pose in chair yoga:

Preparation:

Sit with out problems on a strong chair at the side of your ft flat on the floor, hip-width apart.

Place your hands in your thighs or knees, palms going through down, in a comfortable and open posture.

Ensure your backbone is right away, and your shoulders are comfortable.

Chair-Assisted Triangle Pose:

Step 1: Find Your Foundation:

Begin with the useful resource of sitting without problems on the chair collectively along side your feet flat at the floor.

Imagine your sitting bones rooted firmly into the chair seat, growing stability.

Step 2: Prepare Your Leg Position:

Start together with your right leg. Inhale deeply as you improve your right foot off the ground.

Extend your right leg immediately out to the proper, maintaining it parallel to the ground.

Your ft need to aspect beforehand.

Step 3: Find Your Balance:

While retaining your left foot flat at the floor, pivot your right foot to the proper.

Your toes should point to the component, and your proper heel want to be aligned at the side of your left heel.

Imagine a line connecting your proper heel for your left heel, developing a right away line collectively together together with your chair.

Step 4: Extend Your Right Arm:

Inhale deeply as you enlarge your right arm overhead, reaching it inside the path of the proper.

Keep your palm handling down and your palms prolonged.

Step 5: Lean to the Left:

Exhale slowly as you lean your higher body to the left, far from your proper leg.

Reach your left arm down the left leg, aiming to preserve your hand to the chair seat or shin.

Keep your proper arm prolonged and your gaze up in the course of your right hand.

Step 6: Hold and Breathe:

Take gradual, deep breaths as you maintain the Chair-Assisted Triangle Pose.

Focus on the stretch alongside your proper aspect and the engagement of your leg muscle tissues.

Step 7: Release and Switch Sides:

Inhale as you come back to an upright function, reducing your proper arm to your component.

Chapter 10: Balance And Core Strengthening

Seated Leg Lifts in Chair Yoga

Seated Leg Lifts are a easy but effective chair yoga exercise that dreams the muscles to your legs, in particular the quadriceps, hamstrings, and hip flexors. This exercise is appropriate for people of all health degrees and may assist decorate decrease body strength, flexibility, and move. Here's the way to carry out Seated Leg Lifts in chair yoga:

Preparation:

Sit effortlessly on a robust chair collectively with your feet flat on the floor, hip-width aside.

Place your hands in your thighs or knees, hands handling down, in a snug and open posture.

Ensure your spine is straight away, and your shoulders are comfortable.

Seated Leg Lifts:

Step 1: Find Your Foundation:

Begin with the useful resource of sitting together collectively together with your lower back towards the chair's backrest and your ft flat at the ground.

Imagine your sitting bones rooted firmly into the chair seat, growing stability.

Step 2: Lift One Leg:

Inhale deeply as you elevate your right foot off the ground, keeping your knee bent at a 90-diploma mind-set.

Extend your right leg earlier, elevating it to a cushty pinnacle. It does not want to be very high; the cause is to engage your leg muscle tissues.

Step three: Point and Flex Your Foot:

While maintaining your proper leg inside the lifted role, element your ft ahead, stretching your calf muscular tissues.

Then, flex your foot via pulling your toes decrease again within the path of your shin, attractive your shin muscular tissues.

Perform this pointing and flexing movement numerous times to promote ankle flexibility and movement.

Step four: Lower Your Leg:

Exhale as you lower your right leg decrease lower back to the ground, setting your foot flat.

Take a 2nd to rest and reset your posture.

Step five: Repeat with the Other Leg:

Inhale deeply as you raise your left foot off the ground, maintaining your knee bent at a ninety-degree mindset.

Extend your left leg beforehand, elevating it to a cushty pinnacle.

Point and flex your left foot as you in all likelihood did with the proper foot.

Exhale as you lower your left leg all over again to the ground.

Step 6: Continue Alternating:

Repeat the leg lifts, alternating among your right and left legs.

Aim for 10-15 repetitions on every leg or as many as you experience cushty doing.

Step 7: Breathe Mindfully:

Focus for your breath all through the workout, breathing in as you lift your leg and exhaling as you lower it.

Keep your movements sluggish and managed, preserving recognition of the sensations for your legs.

Tips:

Keep your lower back right away and your center engaged to help your posture in the course of the exercising.

Start with small leg lifts and regularly increase the height as your power and versatility decorate.

If you've got any medical situations or barriers, communicate over collectively with your healthcare company or a chair yoga teacher earlier than trying Seated Leg Lifts.

Seated Leg Lifts in chair yoga offer a handy and effective way to enhance your leg muscle groups, improve flexibility, and boom circulate while seated in a snug and available characteristic. Incorporating this workout into your regular can make a contribution to better decrease body strength and normal well-being.

Knee to Chest in Chair Yoga

Knee to Chest is a slight and on hand chair yoga pose that offers a relaxing stretch for the decrease again and permits launch anxiety in the hips and decrease backbone. This pose is mainly beneficial for human beings with lower again pain or stiffness. Here's a way to carry out Knee Chest chair yoga:

Preparation:

Sit quite without a doubt on a robust chair together with your feet flat on the floor, hip-width apart.

Place your arms to your thighs or knees, palms coping with down, in a cushty and open posture.

Ensure your spine is directly, and your shoulders are relaxed.

Knee to Chest:

Step 1: Find Your Foundation:

Begin via manner of the usage of sitting efficiently on the chair in conjunction with your ft flat on the ground.

Imagine your sitting bones rooted firmly into the chair seat, growing stability.

Step 2: Start with Your Right Leg:

Inhale deeply as you deliver your right foot off the ground, bending your knee.

Hold your right knee with both fingers, interlocking your arms just below the kneecap.

Step three: Hug Your Knee to Your Chest:

Exhale slowly as you gently pull your proper knee within the course of your chest.

Keep your left foot flat on the floor for assist.

As you do that, you have to enjoy a cushty stretch to your proper hip and reduce once more.

Step four: Hold and Breathe:

Hold the placement for some deep breaths, permitting the stretch to deepen with each exhale.

Focus on the sensation of releasing anxiety for your decrease again and hip.

Step five: Release Your Right Leg:

Inhale as you slowly launch your proper knee and decrease your proper foot lower lower back to the floor.

Take a second to relaxation and reset your posture.

Step 6: Repeat with Your Left Leg:

Inhale deeply as you deliver your left foot off the floor, bending your knee.

Hold your left knee with each hands, interlocking your hands in truth under the kneecap.

Exhale as you lightly pull your left knee closer to your chest, feeling the stretch on your left hip and decrease lower back.

Hold for a few deep breaths.

Step 7: Release and Reset:

Inhale to release your left knee and lower your left foot to the floor.

Sit absolutely for a second, allowing the advantages of the stretch to settle in.

Tips:

Perform the Knee to Chest pose with slow, managed movements to avoid any soreness or pressure.

If you have got lower lower back issues or limited flexibility, you can alter this pose via lifting your knee to a comfortable top instead of hugging it tightly to your chest.

If you've got have been given any medical situations or obstacles, talk over together with your healthcare corporation or a chair yoga trainer in advance than attempting Knee to Chest.

Knee-to-chest in-chair yoga is a mild manner to relieve tension in the lower once more and hips, making it an notable desire for the ones searching for to ease ache or stiffness. Regular workout of this pose can contribute to stepped forward flexibility inside the hips and decrease backbone, promoting a more experience of relaxation and well-being.

Seated Boat Pose (Navasana) in Chair Yoga

Seated Boat Pose, or Navasana, is a changed version of the traditional Boat Pose, tailored for chair yoga. This variant lets in people with restricted mobility or balance issues to experience the middle-strengthening and belly-firming benefits of the pose. The seated Boat Pose allows beautify center energy, stability, and posture on the identical time as very last seated. Here's the way to carry out Seated Boat Pose in chair yoga:

Preparation:

Sit with no trouble on a robust chair collectively along with your toes flat on the ground, hip-width apart.

Place your arms in your thighs or knees, palms dealing with down, in a comfortable and open posture.

Ensure your backbone is instantly, and your shoulders are comfortable.

Seated Boat Pose in a Chair:

Step 1: Find Your Foundation:

Begin with the useful resource of using sitting quite surely at the chair together together with your toes flat at the floor.

Imagine your sitting bones rooted firmly into the chair seat, growing balance.

Step 2: Engage Your Core:

Inhale deeply as you've got interplay your middle muscles through lightly pulling your navel within the route of your spine.

This engagement will offer balance for the pose.

Step three: Lift Your Legs:

Exhale slowly as you enhance every of your ft off the ground, maintaining your knees bent.

Aim to carry your thighs parallel to the ground, developing a "V" shape together along with your torso and thighs.

Your shins should be more or less parallel to the floor.

Step 4: Balance:

Find your stability on this function, ensuring that you're feeling stable and sturdy.

Keep your hands for your thighs or knees for manual if wished.

Step 5: Extend Your Arms:

Inhale deeply as you extend your arms clean, parallel to the floor.

Keep your fingers handling each unique and your fingers unfold sizable.

Step 6: Hold and Breathe:

Take sluggish, deep breaths as you keep the Seated Boat Pose.

Focus on attractive your center and preserving your stability.

Step 7: Release:

Exhale as you decrease your toes decrease lower back to the ground, returning to a seated characteristic.

Relax and take some deep breaths to recover.

Tips:

Start with small lifts and step by step artwork closer to lifting your feet better as your core strength improves.

If you have trouble lifting each feet, you could begin via lifting one foot at a time.

If balancing is hard, you can use the backrest of the chair for aid.

Seated Boat Pose in Chair yoga gives a valuable possibility to bolster your center muscular tissues, enhance balance, and beautify posture even as last seated in a comfortable and available function. Regular exercising of this pose can make a contribution to better center energy, stability, and state-of-the-art nicely-being.

Chapter 11: Gentle Stretching And Relaxation

Seated Side Stretch in Chair Yoga

Seated Side Stretch is a mild and powerful chair yoga pose that gives a relaxing stretch for the rims of your body, mainly the ribcage, waist, and reduce lower back. This pose enables beautify flexibility, launch anxiety inside the torso, and encourage deep breathing. Here's the way to carry out Seated Side Stretch in chair yoga:

Preparation:

Sit quite in reality on a robust chair together with your toes flat on the ground, hip-width apart.

Place your hands to your thighs or knees, hands managing down, in a cushty and open posture.

Ensure your spine is at once, and your shoulders are comfortable.

Seated Side Stretch:

Step 1: Find Your Foundation:

Begin by way of way of sitting with out hassle on the chair at the side of your feet flat on the ground.

Imagine your sitting bones rooted firmly into the chair seat, developing stability.

Step 2: Inhale and Lift Your Arms:

Inhale deeply as you enhance every palms overhead, carrying out up inside the path of the ceiling.

Keep your palms handling each one-of-a-type and your hands prolonged.

Step 3: Exhale and Lean to One Side:

Exhale slowly as you lean your top frame to the right, growing a moderate arch in your left facet.

Keep your left hip firmly planted at the chair.

Avoid lifting your right hip off the chair seat.

Step four: Reach with Your Right Arm:

Reach your right arm overhead and to the left, developing an extended stretch along your right aspect.

Feel the stretch out of your right hip for your fingertips.

Step 5: Hold and Breathe:

Hold the Seated Side Stretch for a few deep breaths, feeling the increase of your ribcage and the lengthening of your right issue.

Step 6: Inhale and Return to Center:

Inhale as you slowly skip lower again to an upright, centered feature together with your palms overhead.

Take a 2nd to reset and put together for the opportunity aspect.

Step 7: Exhale and Lean to the Opposite Side:

Exhale as you lean your better body to the left this time, developing a mild arch in your right issue.

Keep your proper hip firmly planted on the chair seat, preserving off any lifting.

Step 8: Reach with Your Left Arm:

Lengthen your left facet at the same time as raising your left arm above and to the right.

Feel the stretch from your left hip to your fingertips.

Step 9: Hold and Breathe:

Hold the stretch for some deep breaths, focusing on the growth of your ribcage and the release of hysteria in your torso.

Step 10: Inhale and Return to Center:

Inhale deeply as you come to an upright, targeted characteristic collectively with your arms overhead.

Exhale and reduce your palms on your factors, taking a 2d to loosen up and breathe deeply.

Tips:

Perform the Seated Side Stretch with sluggish, managed actions, and avoid any sudden or jerky motions.

Focus on your breath, breathing in deeply to increase your ribcage and exhaling completely to launch tension.

You can perform this stretch a couple of times on each aspect, depending on your comfort degree.

Seated Side Stretch in chair yoga is an brilliant way to release tension inside the torso, improve flexibility, and encourage deep, aware respiratory. Regular workout of this pose can contribute to higher posture, decreased stiffness, and an not unusual enjoy of rest and properly-being.

Seated Pigeon Pose in Chair Yoga

Seated Pigeon Pose, additionally referred to as Chair Pigeon Pose, is a changed model of the traditional Pigeon Pose, tailored for chair yoga. This version permits human beings with restrained mobility or flexibility to enjoy the advantages of hip starting off and stretching. Seated Pigeon Pose permits alleviate anxiety within the hip joints and decrease another time whilst promoting relaxation. Here's the way to perform Seated Pigeon Pose in chair yoga:

Preparation:

Sit comfortably on a robust chair collectively along with your feet flat at the floor, hip-width aside.

Place your palms in your thighs or knees, fingers going via down, in a snug and open posture.

Ensure your spine is straight away, and your shoulders are relaxed.

Seated Pigeon Pose in a Chair:

Step 1: Find Your Foundation:

Begin via sitting easily at the chair alongside side your feet flat on the floor.

Imagine your sitting bones rooted firmly into the chair seat, growing stability.

Step 2: Cross Your Right Ankle Over Your Left Knee:

Inhale deeply as you enhance your proper foot off the ground.

Make a decide-four collectively together with your legs through crossing your right ankle over your left knee.

Flex your proper foot to shield your ankle and knee.

Step three: Engage Your Core:

Engage your middle muscle mass through manner of gently pulling your navel closer to your backbone to assist your posture.

Step 4: Hug Your Knee Towards Your Chest:

Exhale slowly as you lightly press your proper knee down and in the direction of your chest.

Your right buttocks and hips want to experience stretched.

Step five: Hold and Breathe:

Hold the Seated Pigeon Pose for some deep breaths, allowing the stretch to deepen with each exhale.

Focus on liberating anxiety for your hip and retaining a snug top body.

Step 6: Release and Switch Sides:

Inhale as you release your right foot and location it once more at the ground.

Take a 2d to rest and reset your posture.

Step 7: Cross Your Left Ankle Over Your Right Knee:

Inhale deeply as you boost your left foot off the floor.

Cross your left ankle over your proper knee, growing the determine-four shape collectively at the side of your legs.

To protect your ankle and knee, bend your left foot.

Step 8: Hug Your Knee Towards Your Chest:

Exhale slowly as you lightly press your left knee down and inside the course of your chest.

Feel the stretch for your left hip and buttocks.

Step 9: Hold and Breathe:

Hold the pose for some deep breaths, that specialize in relaxation and deepening the stretch.

Step 10: Release and Return to Center:

Inhale as you release your left foot and region it decrease returned at the floor.

Sit effectively for a 2d, allowing the advantages of the stretch to settle in.

Tips:

Perform Seated Pigeon Pose with slow, managed movements, and keep away from any forceful or sudden motions.

Focus in your breath, breathing in deeply to enlarge your chest and exhaling sincerely to release tension.

You can carry out this stretch a couple of instances on each issue, counting on your comfort diploma.

Seated Pigeon Pose in chair yoga offers an possibility to release anxiety within the hips and reduce again, enhance hip flexibility, and encourage rest whilst remaining seated in a snug and available function. Regular workout of this pose can contribute to better hip mobility, decreased stiffness, and an normal experience of ease and nicely-being.

Guided Relaxation and Breathing Exercises in Chair Yoga

Guided rest and respiratory sporting sports are critical components of chair yoga exercising. They promote strain comfort, rest, and mindfulness, which may be useful for every mental and physical well-being. These bodily sports can be specifically helpful for seniors over 60, as they could decorate basic fitness and decrease the impact of pressure-related situations. Here are some guided relaxation and respiration bodily video games you can include into your chair yoga ordinary:

1. Deep Breathing (Pranayama):

Sit with no trouble to your chair along side your ft flat at the floor.

Take a moment to loosen up your body as you close up up your eyes.

Inhale deeply through your nostril, increasing your stomach and chest as you fill your lungs with air.

Release any anxiety or stress with the aid of taking a gradual, complete exhale.

Continue deep respiration for severa cycles, focusing on the rhythm of your breath.

This exercising calms the anxious device and can be achieved as a standalone exercising or included into your chair yoga session.

2. Progressive Muscle Relaxation:

Start at your toes and paintings your way up via your frame.

For every muscle company, inhale deeply and anxious the muscle groups for some seconds.

Exhale as you release the tension, permitting the muscle tissues to loosen up absolutely.

Move from your feet on your calves, thighs, abdomen, chest, hands, and neck.

This workout promotes relaxation and allows relieve bodily anxiety.

three. Guided Imagery:

Close your eyes and visualize a peaceful and serene vicinity, which incorporates a seaside, wooded area, or meadow.

Imagine your self in this tranquil setting, engaging all your senses. Feel the warmth of the solar, the softness of the sand, or the rustling of leaves.

Spend a couple of minutes immersed on this intellectual get away, letting skip of any issues or stressors.

Guided imagery can transport you to a country of rest and intellectual readability.

four. Mindful Breath Counting:

Sit for your chair along facet your eyes closed.

Exhale via your mouth after taking a large breath through your nose.

Count every breath cycle, beginning with "one" on the inhale and "" at the exhale.

Continue counting your breaths, focusing absolutely at the numbers.

If your mind begins to wander, lightly supply your interest once more to your breath and counting.

This exercise complements interest and mindfulness.

five. Box Breathing:

Inhale deeply through your nostril for a matter of 4.

Hold your breath for a recollect of four.

Exhale slowly and absolutely thru your mouth for a depend of four.

Hold your breath for any other count number of 4 while pausing.

For multiple cycles, repeat this discipline respiration sample.

Box breathing can reduce tension and pressure and create a enjoy of calm.

6. Chair Yoga Nidra:

Sit without troubles on your chair with your eyes closed.

Listen to a guided chair yoga nidra session, that could be a form of guided meditation that induces deep rest.

Follow the teacher's voice as they lead you via a body experiment, breath popularity, and visualization strategies.

Chair yoga nidra is mainly powerful for relaxation and strain discount.

Incorporating this guided rest and respiration carrying sports into your chair yoga exercise can provide a holistic technique to nicely-being for seniors over 60.

These wearing activities promote relaxation, reduce stress, and decorate mindfulness, contributing to advanced highbrow and bodily health. Always carry out the ones sporting occasions at your very very own comfort diploma and go to a healthcare expert when you have any precise fitness problems.

Chapter 12: Chair Yoga Routines

10-Minute Daily Chair Yoga Routine for Seniors Over 60

A 10-minute day by day chair yoga everyday may be an tremendous manner for seniors over 60 to maintain flexibility, mobility, and stylish nicely-being. This routine is designed to be mild, to be had, and effective, helping you start or stop your day on a high-quality check. Here's a simple chair yoga series you may comply with:

1. Seated Mountain Pose (Tadasana):

Put your toes flat at the floor and lighten up for your chair.

To calm yourself down, near your eyes and take a few lengthy, deep breaths.

Reach your fingers overhead, arms coping with each one of a kind, and stretch upward.

Hold for some breaths, feeling the stretch for your spine.

2. Neck and Shoulder Rolls:

Roll your head slowly in a round motion whilst bringing your chin on your chest.

After a few rolls, reverse the direction and roll your head counterclockwise.

Bring your head lower lower again to the middle and roll your shoulders ahead and backward.

three. Wrist and Ankle Circles:

Extend your arms in front of you and rotate your wrists in each instructions.

Lift your feet barely off the ground and make slight circles together collectively along with your ankles in each commands.

This lets in enhance joint mobility on your wrists and ankles.

4. Seated Cat-Cow Stretch:

Sit up proper away and inhale as you arch your once more, lifting your chest and chin.

As you exhale, arch your once more and chin towards your chest.

Repeat this mild flowing movement some times, syncing it together with your breath.

5. Seated Forward Bend (Paschimottanasana):

Straighten your legs within the the front of you as you sit up straight tall.

Inhale as you make bigger your spine, and exhale as you lightly fold ahead from your hips.

Reach your fingers within the direction of your feet or shins, feeling a stretch in your hamstrings and decrease returned.

Hold for a few breaths.

6. Seated Twist (Ardha Matsyendrasana):

Cross your proper leg over your left as you sit up.

Inhale and amplify your spine, and exhale as you lightly twist to the right.

Use your left hand to keep the lower decrease lower back of your chair and your proper hand on your right knee.

Hold the twist for some breaths after which switch components.

7. Seated Pigeon Pose:

Cross your proper ankle over your left knee, flexing your proper foot.

Inhale deeply and sit up, feeling the stretch for your hip.

After a few breaths of maintaining, switch aspects.

eight. Seated Boat Pose (Navasana):

Hold onto the edges of your chair for manual.

Lift both toes off the floor, growing a "V" shape collectively with your legs.

Hold a good core function for a few breaths.

9. Seated Side Stretch:

Sit up tall and reach your right arm overhead, leaning to the left.

Feel the stretch along your right factor.

After some breaths of maintaining, switch additives.

10. Guided Relaxation and Breathing:

Take a while to unwind with the aid of way of closing your eyes.

Practice deep breathing or guided relaxation for a few minutes.

Focus on freeing tension and finding calmness.

Final Thoughts: This 10-minute each day chair yoga normal is a mild way to sell flexibility, reduce stiffness, and beautify rest. It can be with out troubles incorporated into your each day habitual, whether or not or not you begin or prevent your day with it.

Remember to concentrate for your body, breathe mindfully, and carry out the actions at a pace that feels snug for you. Over time, steady workout can motive advanced mobility and an advanced feel of nicely-being.

30-Minute Chair Yoga Routine for Seniors Over 60

A 30-minute chair yoga ordinary gives a extra whole workout that lets in seniors over 60 to work on power, flexibility, balance, and relaxation. This habitual can be tailored on your desires and modified for your consolation. Here's a 30-minute chair yoga series to bear in mind:

1. Seated Mountain Pose (Tadasana): (2 mins)

Begin in a seated position on the facet of your feet flat on the floor.

Close your eyes, sit up tall, and take a few deep breaths.

Stretch your arms overhead, fingers managing each exclusive.

Hold the pose for a few breaths to center your self.

2. Neck and Shoulder Rolls: (2 minutes)

Gently roll your head in a clockwise direction, then opposite it counterclockwise.

Roll your shoulders forward and backward.

Relax your shoulders and neck if they may be stressful.

three. Deep Breathing (Pranayama): (3 mins)

Put your feet up, close your eyes, and supply interest on your breathing.

Take a four-depend deep breath through your nostril.

For a depend number variety of six, lightly exhale via your mouth.

Continue deep breathing for a couple of minutes to calm your thoughts.

4. Seated Warm-up Stretches: (5 mins)

Perform mild heat-up stretches, which includes ankle circles, wrist circles, and knee lifts.

Focus on every joint to enhance mobility.

five. Seated Cat-Cow Stretch: (3 mins)

In the "Cow Pose," you exhale while you boom your chest and arch your yet again.

In the "Cat Pose," inhale, round your again, and tuck your chin.

The transition amongst the ones stances should be fluid.

6. Seated Forward Bend (Paschimottanasana): (4 mins)

Straighten your legs in front of you.

Inhale and lengthen your backbone, then exhale as you lightly fold ahead out of your hips.

Reach for your feet or shins, keeping the stretch for numerous breaths.

7. Seated Twist (Ardha Matsyendrasana): (4 minutes)

Cross your proper leg over your left.

As you rotate to the right, inhale, stretch your backbone, after which exhale.

Use your left hand to maintain the again of the chair and your proper hand to your proper knee.

Hold the twist for numerous breaths after which transfer aspects.

8. Seated Leg Lifts: (four mins)

Hold onto the edges of your chair for help.

Lift one leg at a time, straightening it as a good deal as snug.

Alternate amongst legs, engaging your middle.

nine. Chair-Assisted Warrior I and II: (5 minutes)

Use the backrest of the chair for useful resource.

Perform Chair-Assisted Warrior I and Chair-Assisted Warrior II on both facets.

These poses assist with balance and power.

10. Guided Relaxation and Breathing: (2 minutes)

Close your eyes and exercising deep respiratory.

Listen to a guided relaxation or meditation for a few minutes.

11. Seated Pigeon Pose: (3 mins)

Cross one ankle over your opposite knee.

Inhale and sit up straight tall, then exhale as you gently press your knee all the way proper right down to experience the stretch on your hip.

Switch factors.

12. Seated Boat Pose (Navasana): (2 mins)

Hold onto the sides of your chair for aid.

Lift every ft off the floor, developing a "V" shape collectively together with your legs.

Engage your middle and maintain the pose for numerous breaths.

thirteen. Final Relaxation: (3 mins)

Sit simply and close to your eyes.

Take some moments to lighten up your body and popularity for your breath.

Let bypass of any final anxiety and discover a country of calmness.

This 30-minute chair yoga routine presents a properly-rounded exercise that addresses numerous factors of your physical and intellectual well-being.

You can alter the period of each pose or upload variations primarily based completely for your wishes and options. Regular exercise of this routine allow you to maintain and decorate your mobility, stability, and commonplace feel of rest and nicely-being.

Chair Yoga for Stress Relief

Chair yoga is a gentle and handy form of yoga that may be mainly powerful for pressure comfort. It's suitable for humans of all ages and health tiers, which encompass seniors over 60. The workout of chair yoga includes appearing yoga poses and relaxation strategies whilst seated in a chair or the use of a chair for useful resource. Here's how chair yoga can help with strain comfort:

1. Promotes Mindfulness:

Chair yoga encourages you to be without a doubt present in the second. By focusing for your breath and moves, you become more aware and privy to your frame, mind, and emotions.

Mindfulness allows destroy the cycle of rumination and fear, redirecting your interest to the proper right here and now, which can lessen pressure.

2. Relaxation Techniques:

Chair yoga contains relaxation strategies which includes deep respiratory, guided imagery, and contemporary muscle rest.

These techniques set off the relaxation response in your body, which counteracts the strain reaction and promotes a experience of calm.

three. Physical Benefits:

Gentle actions and stretches in chair yoga assist release physical anxiety within the body. As you bypass, you release tightness to your muscular tissues, especially in areas at risk of pressure, which includes the neck, shoulders, and decrease lower back.

Improved flexibility and mobility make a contribution to a more cushty and comfortable physical kingdom.

4. Stress Reduction Through Breath Control:

Chair yoga emphasizes managed and deep respiration strategies, collectively with diaphragmatic respiratory and field breathing.

These practices calm the anxious gadget, lessen anxiety, and decorate your body's potential to manipulate pressure.

five. Boosts Mood:

Physical activity, even in a seated role, releases endorphins, the body's herbal temper enhancers.

The aggregate of slight motion and rest strategies in chair yoga can help decorate your temper and reduce signs and symptoms of despair and anxiety associated with stress.

6. Enhances Sleep Quality:

Stress frequently interferes with sleep cycles and motives insomnia or stressed nights.

Chair yoga can help decorate sleep notable with the aid of way of using calming the mind and enjoyable the frame.

Practicing chair yoga earlier than bedtime may be specifically effective in promoting restful sleep.

7. Increases Body Awareness:

Chair yoga fosters a deeper reference to your frame. As you turn out to be greater aware of bodily sensations and anxiety, you could actively launch stress whilst it arises.

This heightened body attention also permit you to understand pressure triggers and positioned into effect rest techniques as wanted.

8. Accessible and Inclusive:

Chair yoga is adaptable and can be modified to suit your character desires and physical talents. It's an inclusive workout that can be loved with the aid of way of humans with numerous bodily limitations.

Everyone can revel in the advantages of chair yoga, regardless of age or health diploma.

9. Reduces Mental Clutter:

Stress regularly ends in racing thoughts and highbrow muddle. The meditative factors of chair yoga assist calm the mind, permitting you to think extra actually and make higher selections.

10. Encourages Self-Care:

Chair yoga offers an possibility for self-care and self-compassion. Taking the time to engage in a slight and nurturing exercising can be a form of self-love and stress control.

Incorporating chair yoga into your each day or weekly ordinary may be an effective strategy for dealing with pressure and selling standard well-being. Whether practiced on my own or as a part of a larger well being plan, chair yoga offers a practical and on hand way to reduce stress, boom relaxation, and beautify your intellectual and bodily resilience.

Chapter 13: Chair Yoga Modifications

Chair Yoga with Props (Bolsters, Blocks, Straps)

Chair yoga is an adaptable and inclusive exercising that may be greater with using props like bolsters, blocks, and straps. These props may additionally want to make chair yoga extra available, cushty, and effective, mainly for seniors over 60 and those with restrained mobility or bodily disturbing situations. Here's how you can comprise props into your chair yoga practice:

1. Bolsters:

Seat Support: Placing a bolster on the seat of your chair can provide more cushioning and guide for your hips and lower decrease returned. This is specifically beneficial when you have pain or ache in these areas.

Leg Support: You can use a bolster to raise your legs, reducing swelling and promoting motion. This is useful for people with leg or ankle troubles.

2. Blocks:

Foot Elevation: Placing yoga blocks below your feet on the same time as seated can create a mild elevation. This may be beneficial for individuals who need to relieve stress on their lower lower lower back or enhance posture.

Arm Support: Use blocks as armrests in your chair to offer useful aid to your arms in the direction of seated poses. This can assist alleviate shoulder and neck tension.

3. Straps:

Enhanced Stretching: Straps may be used to increase your attain in seated stretches. For example, if you have hassle reaching your toes, a strap will assist you to reach and keep your foot sooner or later of a seated ahead bend.

Improved Posture: Straps may be looped at some point of the backrest of the chair to encourage right posture. This enables hold a right away spine, particularly all through longer chair yoga periods.

Gentle Resistance: Wrapping a strap around your thighs or fingers can upload a mild resistance detail in your chair yoga exercise.

This is useful for strengthening sports activities.

Sample Chair Yoga Sequence with Props:

Here's a simple chair yoga collection that includes props:

1. Seated Mountain Pose with Bolster:

Place a bolster at the seat of your chair for added comfort.

Sit on the side of your toes flat on the floor, palms to your thighs, and near your eyes.

To regain your composure, take some extended breaths.

2. Supported Seated Forward Bend with Strap:

Loop a strap across the chair legs and region your ft on the strap to maintain them at hip-width apart.

Inhale and growth your spine, then exhale and hinge ahead out of your hips, accomplishing in your toes or the strap.

Hold for a few breaths, using the strap to softly deepen the stretch.

3. Elevated Legs with Bolster:

Place a bolster beneath your calves, elevating your legs.

This promotes circulate and may reduce swelling inside the lower extremities.

Sit in reality and loosen up, respiratory deeply.

4. Supported Twisting Pose with Blocks:

Place yoga blocks underneath your hands at the chair seat.

Inhale and extend your backbone, then exhale and lightly twist to the right, the usage of the blocks for guide.

Hold for some breaths, then repeat on the left side.

five. Arm Stretches with Blocks:

Use blocks as armrests for your chair.

Sit up straight away, and as you inhale, deliver your hands overhead.

Exhale and reduce your palms, feeling the stretch for your shoulders.

6. Relaxation with Bolster and Eye Pillow:

Place a bolster in your chair and rest your pinnacle body on it.

Close your eyes and use an eye pillow for brought relaxation.

Take several minutes to loosen up and breathe deeply.

Using props in chair yoga lets in for a deeper, greater supported practice. It's important to modify the props on your specific desires and comfort diploma. Props can help make chair yoga an amusing and healing experience, enhancing your flexibility, balance, and relaxation. If you're new to using props on your exercise, bear in mind running with a chair yoga teacher who can guide you efficiently.

Chair Yoga for Joint Health

Chair yoga is a mild and available shape of yoga that can provide first-rate advantages for joint fitness, specifically for seniors over 60 and people with joint issues or restrained mobility. The workout makes a speciality of slight movements, stretches, and relaxation techniques at the same time as seated in a chair or the usage of a chair for beneficial useful resource. Here's how chair yoga can promote joint health:

1. Improved Range of Motion:

Chair yoga consists of some of joint-great movements that help beautify your joints' range of motion. Regular workout can reduce stiffness and enhance flexibility, making every day sports activities much less difficult.

2. Gentle Strength Building:

Chair yoga consists of poses that engage and deliver a boost to the muscles spherical your joints with out placing immoderate stress on them. This introduced muscle useful resource can protect your joints and enhance stability.

three. Pain Reduction:

Many people experience joint ache because of conditions collectively with arthritis or age-related wear and tear. Chair yoga can help alleviate joint ache with the useful resource of promoting flow into, lowering inflammation, and freeing anxiety.

four. Enhanced Synovial Fluid Circulation:

Synovial fluid is a natural lubricant that nourishes and protects your joints. Chair yoga moves, even though seated, can help stimulate the flow of synovial fluid, retaining your joints nicely-lubricated.

five. Mindful Movement:

Chair yoga emphasizes conscious, managed movements that encourage you to be aware of your body's signals. This mindfulness can help you keep away from overexertion or positions that could strain your joints.

6. Reduced Risk of Injury:

Chair yoga affords a secure and supportive environment for training yoga poses. The chair offers balance and stability, reducing the chance of falls or injuries that would arise during conventional yoga.

7. Improved Circulation:

Chair yoga contains deep respiratory strategies and stretches which could decorate blood go together with the float for your joints. Better circulate can sell joint fitness and reduce the hazard of stiffness.

8. Stress Reduction:

Chronic strain can make a contribution to joint infection and pain. Chair yoga includes relaxation strategies that assist lessen stress, that would indirectly benefit your joint health.

nine. Adaptability:

Chair yoga is instead adaptable and may be tailored to cope with unique joint problems or bodily obstacles. Poses and moves can be modified to suit your comfort degree and desires.

10. Enhanced Body Awareness:

Chair yoga promotes a better relationship along with your frame. As you emerge as extra aware of how your joints enjoy and flow into, you could regulate your exercise to keep away from positions that could worsen joint pain.

Sample Chair Yoga Poses for Joint Health:

Here are some chair yoga poses that might promote joint health:

1. Ankle Circles:

Lift one foot barely off the ground and make mild circles along side your ankle in every commands.

This lets in enhance ankle joint mobility.

2. Knee Extensions:

Sit up at once and make bigger one leg forward, lifting your foot slightly off the floor.

Hold for some breaths after which switch legs.

This exercise promotes knee joint flexibility.

3. Wrist Rolls:

Sit up tall and increase your hands within the front of you.

Make moderate wrist circles in each pointers to alleviate wrist joint tension.

4. Shoulder Shrugs:

Inhale deeply and raise your shoulders towards your ears.

Exhale and launch them down.

Repeat this a few instances to reduce tension in the shoulder joints.

five. Seated Cat-Cow Stretch:

Inhale and arch your again (Cow Pose), and then exhale and spherical your back (Cat Pose).

Flow among those poses improves spinal flexibility and relieves stress at the vertebral joints.

6. Gentle Hip Circles:

Sit with out a problem and make moderate hip circles in each hints.

This allows maintain hip joint mobility and decrease stiffness.

7. Seated Mountain Pose:

Sit with your toes flat on the floor and your fingers resting for your thighs.

Close your eyes and interest for your breath to create a feel of usual joint rest.

Regular practice of chair yoga for joint health can make a contribution to more comfort, flexibility, and mobility, making ordinary sports activities extra possible and interesting. Always are looking for advice from a healthcare expert or an authorized yoga teacher when you have specific joint problems or situations earlier than beginning any exercise software program, together with chair yoga.

Chair Yoga for Pain Management

Chair yoga is an available and powerful exercise for coping with numerous types of pain, which incorporates persistent ache, arthritis, joint pain, and muscle tension. It gives mild movements, stretches, and relaxation strategies at the equal time as seated in a chair or the use of a chair for resource. Here's how chair yoga can assist with ache manage:

1. Gentle Stretching and Movement:

Chair yoga consists of moderate stretches and movements which could alleviate stiffness and muscle tension, which may be often belongings of pain.

2. Improved Flexibility:

Regular chair yoga exercising can enhance flexibility, making it much less tough to transport and decreasing the danger of muscle strain and pain.

3. Enhanced Circulation:

Chair yoga moves and deep breathing strategies sell better blood flow, that can help lessen ache and inflammation.

four. Muscle Relaxation:

The rest techniques in chair yoga can help launch muscle tension and promote relaxation, reducing ache associated with muscle tightness.

5. Mind-Body Connection:

Chair yoga emphasizes mindfulness and cognizance of the frame. This will permit you to higher recognize and manipulate pain triggers.

6. Pain Reduction Through Breathing:

Deep respiratory strategies practiced in chair yoga can spark off the relaxation response on your body, reducing ache perception.

7. Stress Reduction:

Chronic pain is frequently associated with pressure and tension. Chair yoga consists of relaxation sporting activities that may lessen strain, in a roundabout manner alleviating pain.

8. Enhanced Posture:

Maintaining right posture thru chair yoga can alleviate pain within the neck, shoulders, and reduce decrease returned, which frequently consequences from horrible alignment.

9. Joint Health:

Chair yoga poses and moves can enhance joint mobility and decrease pain associated with arthritis or joint ache.

Chapter 14: Tips For A Safe And Effective Practice

Staying Hydrated and Nutrition Tips for Seniors Over 60

Proper hydration and vitamins are important for seniors over 60 to maintain high-quality health, strength levels, and regular well-being. As people age, their our bodies can also moreover enjoy changes in metabolism, digestion, and nutrient absorption, making it even extra important to take note of food regimen and hydration. Here are some hints to help seniors live hydrated and make wholesome dietary choices:

Staying Hydrated:

Make it a dependancy to often consume water sooner or later of the day. Set reminders if vital, as older adults may not continually enjoy thirsty, but their our bodies despite the fact that require hydration.

Choose Hydrating Foods: Foods with high water content material material, which include end result (watermelon, oranges, berries) and veggies (cucumbers, celery, lettuce), can contribute to your each day fluid consumption.

Limit Caffeine and Alcohol: These beverages can cause dehydration. If you consume them, gain this moderately and balance them with water or other hydrating fluids.

Use a Reusable Water Bottle: Carry a reusable water bottle with you to make it smooth to sip water in some unspecified time in the future of the day, whether or no longer you are at domestic or at the skip.

Monitor Medications: Some medicinal capsules also can have diuretic effects, so be privy to any capacity dehydration detail results and regulate your fluid intake for this reason. Consult your healthcare company when you have problems.

Pay Attention to Thirst: Even in case you do now not always experience thirsty, reply for your body's signs and drink at the same time as you do. Dehydration can be honestly detected through thirst.

Eat Hydrating Foods: Soups, broths, and materials with higher water content material can contribute on your everyday hydration.

Nutrition Tips:

Balanced Diet: Aim for a properly-rounded food regimen that consists of a whole lot of food from all food companies. This allows make sure you get essential vitamins and keep a healthful weight.

Portion Control: As metabolism has a tendency to gradual down with age, preserve in thoughts of element sizes to save you overeating. It may be less complicated to govern to devour smaller, extra common food.

Fiber-Rich Foods: Incorporate fiber-rich factors like entire grains, quit end result, veggies, and legumes to guide digestive fitness and modify blood sugar tiers.

Protein Intake: Seniors can also additionally require extra protein to hold muscle companies and strength. Include lean belongings of protein, together with hen, fish, tofu, beans, and nuts, for your eating regimen.

Calcium and Vitamin D: Ensure you are getting ok calcium and nutrients D for bone health. Dairy products, fortified meals, and dietary dietary supplements, if recommended by using way of a healthcare agency, can help.

Limit Sodium: Reduce sodium consumption to govern blood pressure and minimize the danger of coronary heart sickness. Avoid or restrict mainly processed and salty food.

Healthy Fats: Include property of healthful fats, like avocados, nuts, seeds, and olive oil, at the equal time as minimizing saturated and trans fats located in fried and processed components.

Fruits and Vegetables: Aim to fill half of of your plate with cease end result and vegetables to provide essential vitamins, minerals, and antioxidants.